M000208060

PRAISE FOR *STARE BY YOUR MANHOOD*

'It is: intelligent, very well-researched including extensive interviews with many female academics, myth-busting, articulate, witty, upbeat, challenging, surprising, laugh-out-loud funny in places, shocking in others, angry, compassionate, respectful of women, optimistic and a really good read.'
– Huffington Post

'[An] angry, funny, provocative book [that] certainly offers plenty of food for thought. I am stirred by his rallying call for us to become "suffragents".'
– *Daily Mail* (Book of the Week)

'A sophisticated tome for the modern man'
– *Daily Mirror*

'A funny, frank read. I don't think I'll ever look at my manhood in the same way again.'
– Danny Wallace

'Controversial'
– Fox News

STAND BY YOUR MANHOOD

AN ESSENTIAL GUIDE FOR MODERN MEN

PETER LLOYD

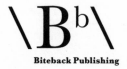

Biteback Publishing

This new edition published in Great Britain in 2016 by
Biteback Publishing Ltd
Westminster Tower
3 Albert Embankment
London SE1 7SP
Copyright © Peter Lloyd 2014, 2016

ISBN 978-1-78590-021-1

10 9 8 7 6 5 4 3 2 1

A CIP catalogue record for this book is available from the British Library.

Set in Adobe Garamond Pro

Printed and bound in Great Britain by
CPI Group (UK) Ltd, Croydon CR0 4YY

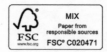

For my mother, Jean, and my father, PJ –

a better team than Everton or Liverpool

CONTENTS

WHY YOU NEED THIS BOOK

MEN ARE BRILLIANT.

Being a man is brilliant. Seriously, it is. Except for penile dysmorphia, circumcision, paying the bill, becoming a weekend father, critics who've been hating on us for, well, pretty much fifty years – oh, and those pesky early deaths.

Suicide isn't much of a laugh either. Nor is paternity

fraud, schools failing boys, military conscription, conception by deception, the criminal sentencing gap, coughing up 70 per cent of income tax, dominating homeless statistics or getting throat cancer from oral sex, which – ironically – is what's really going down for a new, unassuming generation who still aren't briefed on life's nagging bloke truths.

Hence the time is now for a new, improved approach to masculinity.

From our relationships with women to our relations with ourselves, nobody should be more informed on the everyday politics of being men than us. It's our prerogative.

Yet, despite living in society's most liberal age, our greatest ever technological era – where ideas, information and the occasional celebrity porn tape can be shared in an instant – tackling the gritty, salty stuff integral to our well-being, not to mention our hair line, remains strictly off-limits. Not because we can't communicate, but because the truth is inconvenient for everyone else.

Men being honest – really, truly candid about what affects them sexually, financially, legally and psychologically – remains rigidly taboo because it's the ultimate game-changer.

Funnily enough, that's precisely why we should embrace it. Like a piñata for the pissed off, we've spent decades being the trendy target in a long line of public floggings. The overrated, unfashionable gender. The one social group it's politically correct – no, no – *virtuous* to dislike. In fact, man-bashing has become mainstream, so lucrative that people build entire careers on it – which might explain why, for many, it musn't be ruined with a reality check.

The megalomania of it all recently snowballed to the point of censorship, with the European Union attempting to criminalise any criticism of the sisterhood via the (ironically titled) Statute for Promotion of Tolerance, whilst Facebook already suspends users for the same reason – which, together, isn't just bonkers, but a bit Putin, too.

Thankfully, there's light at the end of the tunnel.

When London's Southbank Centre held the UK's first ever men's festival, Being A Man, earlier this year, it was a line in the sand. Putting our issues on the map with a straight-down-the-middle legitimacy, it attracted hundreds of people from all demographics – male, female, young, old, black, white, gay, straight – to chew over the credentials of masculinity in a worthy space. Think Radio 4, but with beards and some really trendy brochure artwork.

Topics ranged from friendship – with Billy Bragg and Phill Jupitus detailing the success of their cast-iron, twenty-year kinship – to mental health, fathers and marriage. Even Tony Blair's former spin doctor, Alastair

Campbell – not to be mistaken for UB40's Ali Campbell, as one onlooker did – detailed his journey back
from alcoholism and depression at a time when men's
self-destruct stats are at a record high.

Aside from being one of the few instances in human
history where men, not women, had to queue for the
toilets, it also offered another first: men were allowed
to dip their toes into feminism – without apology or
the fear of being wrestled into a headlock by Germaine
Greer. About time, too. By this point we'd been criticised
non-stop for about half a century, so were probably due
a right to reply. Maybe even a full-scale comeback, like
the Union Jack. Years ago, it, like us, was considered a
symbol of benevolence and strength, before modern sen-
sitivities made it naff – perhaps even offensive. Although
it never changed, attitudes around it did. So when Mor-
rissey took to the stage in 1992 with it draped across
his shoulders, the *NME* accused him of being racist; an
accusation which, although incorrect, made everyone
edgy. Suddenly, people were fine being patriotic, but only
sheepishly. They didn't possess themselves too loudly for
fear of being misinterpreted as jingoistic and torn down.

It took the Queen's Diamond Jubilee in 2012 for
everybody to finally relax and discover a renewed comfort level with national pride. The reason? They'd been
given permission to.

On some level, Being A Man offered a similar thing. It allowed those wanting to fly the flag of their gender to do so, freely – be it holding doors open, sitting with their legs apart or having a sense of basic worth – without being labelled sexist (or, in the case of *Game of Thrones* actor Richard Madden, threatened with castration).

Although it wasn't perfect, the festival set us off on the long, hard slog of detoxing masculinity and countering the disconnect between us and everything good. Not only did it offer permission for men to be men, but it was also a commercial success – which pricked ears. Since then, similar events have cropped up in India and the US, where, most recently, hundreds gathered in Detroit for America's first conference on men and boys.

Of course, some questioned why they were needed at all. Female critics sneered 'every day is a men's festival', whilst a handful of grandstanding guys asked: 'What's the point of more pale, stale males getting together and talking about themselves?' The answer is simple: because, despite 1.9 million years of evolution, we still haven't *quite* nailed this thing called life.

Even at our best, brilliant people like John Cleese drop the baton – which is disconcerting considering he's one of our better brand ambassadors. Intelligent, acclaimed and in possession of the super-brain behind *Monty Python*, which might just be the funniest sketch show ever, he continually buys into marriage despite three failed attempts, including one to Alyce Faye Eichelberger, who got more of his fortune than he did when they split. Still, after paying her off with £600,000 per year for seven years, an £8 million lump sum, an apartment in New York, a £2 million London mews and half a beach house in California, he soon went off and married somebody else – only signing a last-minute pre-nup on the hair-pulling insistence of lawyers.

Some might call this admirable, but there's nothing romantic about financial ruin.

No less frustrating are the likes of Wimbledon champion Boris Becker, who can ace a sports tournament with ease but can't appreciate that – as a man, and especially a famous, rich man – he's a sitting duck for anyone determined to get a baby with a bursary and a lifestyle to boot. Thus, if he's going to have random sex with an opportunist in a restaurant, he might want to consider the possibility of an ulterior motive, or expect a fax – and a bill – nine months later.

These great men, like millions more, are superlative in countless ways, yet they don't seem to operate at full-truth level. Instead of seeing their vulnerability in the way everybody else does, which would serve them better, they believe their own hype. They take sexual attention at face value. They see strength manifest in their bodies as biceps, triceps and abdominals, or as money in their wallets, and think they're invincible – but they fail to see the personal as political, which means looking at the bigger picture. Joining the dots between individual experience and the larger socio-political structures that bind us.

This, gentlemen, is always the fatal gap in our armour. Not least because women have long been upping their game in this department and their general consensus is that we, as men, deserve bringing down a peg or two.

I once met Caitlin Moran, author of *How To Be a Woman*, during an awards ceremony in London. To her legion of fans she's the voice of contemporary feminism, only funny. Yet, despite her credentials as one of Britain's more well-rounded celebrity 'libbers', she insisted that all men lead a charmed life compared to women – always – which makes positive discrimination against us forever fair game.

The irony of a millionaire explaining this to a lad from Liverpool was not lost on me.

Then again, had I been told this ten years earlier, I might've agreed. After all, that's all we're ever told. Now, however – having burned my briefs – I can see that she's actually only half right. Yes, there are advantages to being male: we can have as much sex as we like without being called slags; we rarely have to worry about being groped on a packed bus or making the Sophie's Choice between kid and career. But we also have our own issues of everyday sexism: denied parental rights; left to die years earlier than women (because NHS spending favours them – as we'll see later); and casually packed off to war like mules. None of this shit is a) power, b) privilege or c) easy.

But if bestselling experts can't see this, it's no wonder men who aren't paid generous sums to discuss gender issues don't either. Ask any man. Or, rather, ask a woman who lived as a man for eighteen months. American journalist Norah Vincent did exactly that as an elaborate premise for her 2006 book *Self-Made Man*. A bridge between two worlds, it gave a unique insight into our lives – and, to her surprise, the experience was every bit as complex, as difficult and as demanding as being a woman.

Specifically, she said:

> It was hard being a guy. Really hard. And there were a lot of reasons for this, most of which, when I recount them, make me sound like a tired and prototypical angry young man. It's not exactly a pose I relish. I used to hate that character … I always found him tedious and unsympathetic. But after living as a guy for even just a small slice of lifetime, I can really relate to that screed and give you one of my own. In fact, that's the only way I can truthfully characterise my life as a guy. I didn't like it…

> I thought that by being a guy I would get to do all the
> things I didn't get to do as a woman, things I'd always
> envied about boyhood when I was a child: the perceived
> freedoms … But when it came to the business of being
> [a man] I rarely felt free at all.

If only the world had listened sooner we could've saved her a job. But, of course, they didn't. They never do. It's almost like the truths of masculinity have become a classified document in recent years – unfit for public consumption. Just like airline companies won't serve energy-generating food on long flights in case they create restless, demanding passengers, the establishment won't share the reality of men's lives: the underbelly of the beer belly.

Instead, they keep us socially sedated with an airbrushed version. Usually one that features a great big pair of tits. Open any bestselling men's magazine and see for yourself. There'll be little evidence of the burning issues we face as a gender. You'll find fast cars, sports stars and women who forgot to get dressed. You'll learn how to cook a steak, 101 ways to please your girlfriend and what to wear whilst asking your wife's permission to get the snip. You know, the really important stuff. It might go on to discuss business, killer six-packs or even the gentrification of the denim shirt, but for a new generation of men this is no longer enough. Because although it's glossy, it's exciting and it entertains – often brilliantly – it also keeps us asleep.

Paradoxically, few of us end up living the dream.

Over the past decade, scores of men have realised that the big-breasted nirvana they saw in *FHM* during the 1990s doesn't really exist. In its place are divorce courts, absent children and prostate trouble. That's not to say these lads' mags don't have their place – they do, because they cheer male sexuality when it's an easy target – but they still don't illustrate the light and shade of reality. And, if knowledge is power, then such editorial engineering, no matter how well meaning, leaves us all a bit, well, impotent.

To be fair, it's partly our own fault. American comedian Bill Burr put it best when he said we don't want to question our gender roles and our relationships with women because we want to fuck them. And he's right. That's why editors talk to our penises, not our brains. However, whilst this approach might get us laid, it's also getting us shafted. Because every man who isn't prudent about his life invites misandry (learn this word – it's the male equivalent of misogyny). Think of it like professional boxing without bobbing and weaving, parrying or being cross-armed in the ring. You'd be performing at a massive disadvantage for no good reason. Yet, as men, we do this all the time in life. And, just like a blind-siding punch, old age or a credit card bill, misandry creeps up on us. It ends up being the eye-watering family law ruling which forces you to become a second-Sunday father – a McDad – or a gold-digger's cash-point. These are the truths that are too ugly for handsome magazines. Trust me, I've worked on them.

They're the same truths that newspapers and top-ranking websites frequently avoid reporting in case they upset the establishment – or worse, their female readership. After all, that'd be bad for business. Most newspapers devote entire sections to women and their well-being because they're the main target of advertising revenue. Men are simply given sports pages and told to be happy.

Journalistically, it's as if we're allowed to discuss the heavy-duty issues like war and politics, but not the war and politics of being male. Granted, some might say the reverse – that the very existence of women-specific supplements separates them – but the reality is that there's little they can't say in them. No women's issues are truly off the agenda, with no insult too offensive. Meanwhile, we're shushed and shamed into compliance. And herein lies our problem: if the women's movement has freed up women, men need their own equivalent. After centuries of succeeding for the mutual benefit of everyone – a bit of anaesthetic here, a spot of rocket science there

– we've spent recent history feeling guilty for it. Instead of having a sense of pride (one that points and laughs when someone says we can't multi-task or use a washing machine, even though we created the damn thing), we now concern ourselves with appearing asexual, being modest and 'finishing last'.

This, we are constantly told, is the new formula for being a man. Succeeding to the point of being useful, but not leading. Or, if we do lead, feeling bad for it. Remembering that if we ever do triumph it's because our achievements are handed to us on a plate, probably at the expense of women, not because we're skilled and work hard.

Suspiciously, this formula misses a sole, independent sense of self that sees men determine for themselves what masculinity is. One that's free of women's approval and isn't dogged by fears of whether she's faking it. Which begs one very important question: is this a *Sex and the City* version of being a man – one that hangs our identity on a thumbs-up from the opposite sex – or is it the real thing?

Fortunately, there's a better acid test to determine our credentials as modern men. And it's this: on top of DIY, Sunday-league football and being able to evict unwelcome spiders, can we rationally, respectfully, intellectually defend the brotherhood when it's under fashionable attack – even if our voice shakes? Because if we cannot, who can – and who will?

Those who don't generally sell out for sex. And although this sounds good, it rarely ends well. Just ask bestselling author Esther Vilar. In 1971, she wrote her trailblazing book *The Manipulated Man*. In it she noted that, contrary to popular belief, women in industrialised countries aren't simply oppressed by all men, all the time, but – rather – it cuts both ways. We manipulate each other. Upon publication she received death threats from 'Gal-Qaeda' extremists – or is it Shehadists? – all over the world, proving that it's not always easy to stand your ground, even if you're making a fair point. Nineteen years later, when Neil Lyndon wrote *No More Sex War* in 1992, a virtual peace treaty between the genders which suggested feminism needed to soften and consider men as allies, not aggressors, little had changed. In fact, the hostility was so irrational that one critic from the *Sunday Times* suggested he must've been motivated by a small penis complex. Charming.

But as Winston Churchill once said, 'You have enemies? Good. That means you've stood up for something, sometime in your life.' And his words remain true. Almost five decades after her book hit the shelves, Vilar said in reflection: 'If I had known then what I know today, I probably wouldn't have written this book.

And that is precisely the reason why I am so glad to have written it.'

Amazingly, after decades of so-called solution feminism, virtually everything in it remains unchanged.

> Men are conscripted; women are not. Men are sent to fight in wars; women are largely not. Men retire later than women (even though, due to their lower life expectancy, they should have the right to retire earlier). Men have almost no influence over their reproduction (for males there is neither a pill nor abortion – they can only get the children women want them to have). Men support women; women never, or only temporarily, support men. Men work all their lives; women work only temporarily or not at all … Men only borrow their children; woman can keep them.

Naturally, this is all our fault. In 2013, British Labour MP Diane Abbott made a damning speech about Britain's men and boys – smugly announcing that masculinity was 'in crisis'. The shadow Public Health Minister – who, rather brilliantly, was later sacked from the front bench by Ed Miliband after failing to toe the party line – declared that male culture is 'a celebration of heartlessness; a lack of respect for women's autonomy and the normalisation of homophobia'. Even for the millions of men who are gay, apparently.

She added that men 'find themselves voluntarily creating an extended adolescence' by living at home with their parents – which has absolutely *nothing* to do with rising house prices, but everything to do with being 'resentful of family life'.

The speech, which made no reference to women's identikit behaviour, might've been funny if it weren't so tragic, so I couldn't help but address it when we met at a charity fundraiser in the V&A museum. There, she admitted that her entire theory came from a chat with a 'handful' of male friends. Hardly a credible, detailed study. Fortunately, the one good thing her rant did do was get people talking. Years ago, such a speech would've gone unchallenged in a bid to be seen to 'get' feminism. But contemporary conversations are a tad more balanced now. The erudite Tony Parsons, who is a total lad, made a blistering retort in his *GQ* column, whilst actor Jude Law told me at the Groucho Club that 'men are no more in crisis than women'. Very true. You see, men don't need focus because they're faltering, but because parity is a two-way street. Thus, if air-brushed images of models make young girls feel bad, then articles entitled 'Why Are Middle-Class Men Useless?' by Janice Turner are crushing for boys. Yet that exact headline appeared on the front page of *The Times*.

This kind of stiletto sexism – popularised by the likes

of Julie Burchill, Suzanne Moore, Rachel Johnson and Barbara Ellen – isn't traditionally something men have had to deal with, so they let it go, hoping it'll pass. But here's a secret I'm willing to share: it hasn't and it won't. Hence this book.

If you become a father to twins – one girl, one boy – current data proves that your son will die younger, leave school with fewer qualifications and be less eligible for work than your daughter.

Statistically, she'll graduate university, but your son will be lucky to make it past the application stage. FYI, women now dominate further education at a rate of one million for 700,000 men, with one London university, the Royal Veterinary College, formally identifying white guys as an under-repesented group. In fact, across the Russell Group of institutes – Birmingham, Bristol, Cambridge, Edinburgh, Glasgow, Imperial College London, Leeds, Liverpool, London School of Economics, Manchester, Newcastle, Nottingham, Oxford, Sheffield, Southampton, University College London and Warwick – only three have a majority of male students.

This means your son will more likely join the ranks of the unemployed … the majority of whom are now – yep, you guessed it – men. The Office of National Staistics noted that, for May–July 2014, 1,147,511 British men were out of work compared to 887,892 women.

The same is happening in the USA, where 80 per cent of the 5.7 million jobs lost by Americans during the financial crisis between December 2007 and May 2009 were held by men. The same men who, at eighteen, were forced to sign up for military service – risking death and injury – or face five years in jail or a $250,000 fine. Currently, non-compliance makes all men ineligible for various federal benefits including employment, financial aid, citizenship, loans, voting and job training – men, but not women.

Psychologically, your son will be more likely to suffer from depression and attempt suicide than his sibling, but there'll be less support in place to save him. More than ten men a day kill themselves in England and Wales; it's by far the biggest cause of death for young men in the UK. If he survives this temptation, he's more likely to endure everyday violence than women, with the Crime Statistics for England and Wales 2011/12 noting that two-thirds of homicide victims were men. The same report also recorded 800,000 cases of domestic violence against males, but awareness campaigns and shelters still only target females. This isn't a simple oversight, but an entire culture that's been cultivated for years.

A lack of respect in wider society will make gang culture appealing, but your son will be blamed for wanting affirmative peers when he joins one. He'll then spend years worrying over his body and sexual ability, because he'll be told that penis size matters, whereas your daughter will be told she's beautiful in every guise. Then, if he's seduced by his female teacher, she'll leave court with a slapped wrist thanks to a legal system which is frequently lenient with women (see the Everyday Bullshit chapter), but if your daughter has an affair with her male maths tutor he'll be chalking up numbers on a prison wall.

By the time your son's eighteen he will probably believe you're less valuable than your wife in terms of parental need – that fathers in families are an added bonus, not a crucial cog. Then, when he grows up, he might start his own family – maybe or maybe not by choice – but if his relationship doesn't last, he'll become one of the four million UK men who have no access to their children, but are forced to fund them.

To cap it all, he'll be progressively neglected by British healthcare, despite being more likely to get – and die from – cancer. Yet NHS funding will pump more money into women's healthcare than men's. Oh, and if he sits next to a child on a commercial airline such as Virgin or British Airways, he'll be moved in case he sexually abuses them. Your daughter won't, even if she has previous form.

At best, a lifetime of this leaves our boys deflated, dispirited and disenfranchised. At worst, it pathologises them. It encourages a suspicion of our sons and nephews, sealing their fate before they've even started. It also tells women they're justified in holding a lazy, dim view of us and can forever do no wrong.

Sadly, like most guys, he'll accept this because, historically, it's what we do. In a bid to support women's emancipation, in a bid for peace, in a bid to maximise our chances of getting laid, we say nothing – we allow jokes to be made about our intellectual ability, our emotional intelligence and our capacity for commitment, without saying a word. But it hasn't worked. The gender war is still a bloody mess.

One reason for this is that nobody ever taught our sons to be part of the balance. Instead, they're told that men who complain should be seen and not heard. Written off as misogynists for daring to demand a fair deal.

Obviously, this isn't to say that girls are off having a fine time – most of society is well-versed on the problems and pressures faced by women. The same women who have spent years trying to prove their worth beyond motherhood and housework. In the Oppression Olympics they'd be Usain Bolt. But, unlike us, they get column inches. They get government funding and MPs. They have a vocal community who will stand in their defence. Specifically, they don't have men telling them to 'woman up'.

Fortunately, since the advent of the internet – a place no editors or agendas can censor – men have re-discovered their footing. Websites and organisations such as the National Coalition For Men and the appropriately titled A Voice for Men have articulated the scope of our issues better than any left-leaning broadsheet ever could (or would), which explains why thousands of 18–24-year-olds visit them every day. Reassuringly, they're not just a bunch of angry, hairy blokes. The editor-at-large of AVFM is Erin Pizzey – the woman who set up the world's first ever domestic violence shelter in London's Chiswick in 1971. Her story, which includes fleeing the country after receiving death threats from hard-liners, is so fascinating that actress Kate Beckinsale, who grew up nearby, now wants to transform it into a Hollywood screenplay. Poignantly, Erin described her role on the site as 'coming home'.

In the Alexa ratings, the system that measures web traffic and online popularity, both are already up there and growing, fast. Why? Because they're bucking a trend where men's magazines aren't. They're telling it straight.

When Sharon Osbourne used American television show *The Talk* to describe Catherine Kieu Becker's attack on her California husband as 'quite fabulous', she got more than she bargained for. Whilst they laughed and cheered the woman who drugged her partner's food with sleeping pills, tied him to a bed, cut his penis off and destroyed it in a garbage disposal unit so it couldn't be re-attached – all because she objected to his request for a divorce – men plagued the network with complaints until Osbourne was forced to apologise. Even one of the cameramen refused to film the live scenes and walked away, leaving producers in a prime-time crisis. Never before had women on US TV been held accountable in such a way. It was genius.

Here in Britain, Fathers 4 Justice have long been modern-day, male equivalents of the suffragettes with their bid to equalise family law, dressing up as superheroes and throwing themselves in front of the proverbial horse.

Together, this all happened with people power – something we'll personally need to be our own propellor of change. After all, nobody's going to do it for us. We are not of interest to MPs, UN panels or charities, so we need to get off the sofa – even just mentally – and help ourselves. Don't panic, I'm not suggesting we take to the streets with placards, but turn on any TV channel or radio station and there's a global conversation about men – sometimes disguised as being about women – taking place without us. These all slowly influence our worlds, which is precisely why we need a male equivalent of feminism: something that will define, defend and expand social equality for blokes and boys, too.

You can be forgiven for laughing at this point because people assume the suggestion is absurd – that such a thing doesn't need to exist, or already does on such a huge scale that it's the natural order of things – but they're wrong. As this book will prove.

But first, we must name it to claim it. Previously, people tried to introduce terms like 'masculinist' to define a bit of well-intended brief-burning, but they never quite stuck – in part because people couldn't actually say them. So what's left – a men's human rights activist? Nah. Too dry. An equalist? Too pious. A feminist? Afraid not – after all, that's incomplete. In the decades that feminism has been the political and social standard it hasn't touched the sides of men's issues, except in ways where it has also helped women (paternity leave is only a top topic for this reason – we're expected to be equal caregivers, but not equal in the law).

Instead, I reckon we should all become Suffragents – a new breed of sane, sorted men whose political interests are jointly at the fore with women's. Not to undo or compete with feminism, but to sit alongside it and create symmetry.

And this, right here, is your formal invitation to be part of it.

Thankfully, more than ever, we are already galvanising in this way, whether consciously or not. Look at Movember. A self-made men's movement, it's been raising consciousness, as well as smiles, since catching the world's imagination in 2003. From the humble beginnings of thirty Australian men fundraising for a dying friend, it's moved in from the fringe of internet ideas to become a major weapon in winning. Still, its Burt Reynolds brilliance isn't just because it has generated more than £345 million across twenty-one countries, bank-rolling 800 programmes and saving countless lives, but because it laughed in the face of people who thought men wouldn't have the collective balls to do it.

Then again, at the opposite end of the scale, it's hard to imagine there was also a time when men didn't use a moisturiser – that the multi-million-pound industry fronted by some of Hollywood's leading figures, including Gerard Butler and Clive Owen, once didn't exist. My point? Things change. The parameters of what's socially acceptable for men shift. Years ago, skincare was for girls, just like feminism. But, in a changing world, men have branded their own version of the same product and included it in their daily routine. The same is happening with man politics: the age of putting up and shutting up is dead.

Eventually, with regular use, this approach will change the face of men's issues, which – whether you like it or not – are *your* issues: Should we fund the first date? Are we sexist if we enjoy pornography? Why are we still waiting for a male pill? And do women secretly hate us? Finally, the answers are all here, in this politically incorrect, yet factually correct, compendium of no-bullshit masculinity for a modern age.

After all, we are brilliant. So let's keep it that way.

THE POLITICS
OF THE PENIS

NO MAN IS EVER BORN with a sense of insecurity about his penis – ever. It's something he's taught.

Fortunately, once you understand this, you can 'un-learn' the toxic myth that size is king and finally be at peace with your penis. Not only is this psychologically healthy, but it also sets you free from a lifetime of put-downs, painful operations and expensive scams which never, ever work.

Best of all, it also makes you bulletproof in the face of size slurs, which are part of everyday life for all men, regardless of how big they actually are.

It hasn't always been this way. In ancient Europe, less was considered more – see Michelangelo's Renaissance masterpiece *David* if you need a visual aid. Today, however, it's a little different – and not just in art. Now, men are rated, denigrated and humiliated by their penises in every facet of life.

For most of us, this a universal experience. One which every bloke, every boy, will have a memory of, neatly tucked away and rarely – if ever – referenced. But it sits there, smirking. I've seen it myself. In some of the most prolific media operations in the country, I've watched smart, clever women in positions of power sell out to stiletto sexism with a hooked little finger, even though any man would be fired if he claimed a female CEO was rude because she had a roomy vulva.

Thankfully, the unspoken truth is that every penis is perfectly fine exactly as it is – including yours. It does not need enlarging, pumping, piercing, widening, trimming, straightening or stiffening. You wouldn't be loved more, better in bed or more popular if it were the size of a fire hose. You'd just be you – exactly who you are now, warts and all – with a few more centimetres. Besides, cock-mocking isn't really about rating length or girth, but about the power that can be gained simply by doing it.

Thankfully, your masculinity, your dignity, your credibility is bigger than that. Chances are, so is your penis. And, even if you think it isn't, size doesn't matter because your best sexual organ is your brain. Read that paragraph again.

In a world where belittling men's bodies is often confused with women's sexual literacy, this is important to remember. Currently, despite their life-creating brilliance, our dicks face regular ridicule in everything from song lyrics to government road safety campaigns. (No, really – thank Australia for that one. In 2007, Sydney's Road and Traffic Authority ran the 'Pinkie' ad 'Speeding: No One Thinks Big of You', which showed women equating reckless driving with smaller genitalia.)

Here in Britain, we have Lily Allen doing it for them. She spends hours slagging off MailOnline for 'judging' women's bodies and putting pressure on the sisterhood to be a certain size and shape (even though it's mostly female journalists who write these articles, and female readers, including her, who consume them), but she doesn't extend the same courtesy to lads.

First she released 'Not Big', in which she muses about her classy size demands by singing: 'You're not big, you're not clever, No, you ain't ya big brother. I'm gonna tell the world you're rubbish in bed. And that you're small in the game.' Lovely. Then, Goldicock's second family-friendly offering was 'Not Fair', which sees her deride a boyfriend for not giving her an orgasm when, where and how she demands it. The lyrics are: 'Oh, he treats me with respect, he says he loves me all the time … There's just one thing that's getting in the way. When we go up to bed, you're just no good … It's not fair and I think you're really mean.'

Now, I don't want to get into the nitty gritty of Lily's sex life – in fact, I can't think of anything worse – but wow: isn't this the pot calling the kettle black? Here we have a prime example of a woman who says making people feel bad about their bodies is cruel and harmful, sexist even, yet she does exactly that. Unsurprisingly, when I call her out about this on Twitter it instantly hits a nerve. She responds within seconds, arguing that the songs are about 'specific men, not all men', so she's 'not a hypocrite'.

I can only imagine how comforting that is for her ex-boyfriends, not to mention her son who, in case she hasn't noticed, has a penis.

But what would happen if a singer like Ed Sheeran or Paolo Nutini released a track about the equivalent – a specific woman, an ex, who needed to do more Kegel exercises at the bus stop? Or a former lover dumped because it was like throwing a sausage down

Oxford Street? We all enjoy a bit of good-natured, self-deprecating humour – after all, none of us are perfect and the human form exerts a fascination with all its quirks – but it wouldn't get airplay and it certainly wouldn't be considered funny. Christ, it wouldn't even get released. So what's the difference?

See, whilst dick-dissing is portrayed as good fun for girls, the reality is considerably darker because, actually, Ms Allen is spot on. All this negativity *does* coalesce in peoples' minds and, if they're not thick-skinned enough to handle it, it can damage them. It sparks a chain reaction. Boys start worrying about their dicks, then start acting like dicks. They strap on 'elongating' devices which promise to stretch them if they wear it for ten hours every day of the year at the bargain price of £1,000. Or they try the Middle Eastern technique 'jelqing', which can only be described as trying to stretch a jumper after you've put it in the dryer.

Not only does this make me wince with sympathy pains, but I dread to think what happens when these guys invest all their time and money, but see absolutely no difference at the end of it. One thing's for sure, they wouldn't get any sympathy from the outside world: we're fair game.

When Jude Law was photographed naked on holiday at his mother's private villa in France, the media couldn't resist printing the shots, with the suggestion that every redeeming quality about him – his talent, his good looks, his success, his intelligence, his skills as a father – had all been deleted because in his trousers was an utterly NORMAL penis.

In an article entitled 'Nude Jude's Not A Huge Issue', the *New York Post* wrote: 'In snapshots that recall George Costanza's infamous "shrinkage" episode on *Seinfeld*, the love-rat actor's meager manhood is on full display as he changes into a swimsuit outside his mother Maggie Law's house in Vaudelnay, France.' Meanwhile, Gawker (check out the hypocrisy of their strict moral code in the Sex Isn't Sexist chapter) chimed in: 'Photos of Jude Law's peniwinkle have been circulating. It'd be cruel for us not to share them with you. So, make sure your boss isn't looking, click here to see the itty bitty fella, roll eyes, take [a] shower [and] get circumcising.'

Then again, should we really be surprised? Even Napoleon's penis wasn't sacred. Removed during his autopsy, it later went on display in a New York exhibition, where *Time* magazine said it resembled a 'shriveled eel'. Half a century later and the staff at *Elle* – who collectively couldn't achieve half of what he did, even with the advantage of everything men have created since – are still banging on about his alleged 'tiny scepter'.

Yet when Kate Middleton was papped sunbathing

topless, everyone was furious. Violation! Sexist! Rude! I wanted to weep. Not because of Jude's genitals, which were perfectly fine, but because our private parts are forever ridiculed in a way women's aren't. OK, breasts adorn page three, but at least they're celebrated. They're not put up to be laughed at. Ours are. Even multinational companies like Pepsi, who sell their soft drinks to children, for God's sake, use slogans such as 'Size Does Matter', which isn't just offensive, but really shit copywriting. I can do better on the back of a fag packet. Drunk.

Most people justify this by saying it only affects arrogant men, who somehow deserve it. On the contrary, I'd bet a small fortune the blokes taking the biggest blows are those battling a depressing size neurosis. Once, a seventeen-year-old boy emailed me via my website. He'd quit his rugby team, stopped going out and refused to date girls – all because he thought his penis wasn't 'good enough'. He also refused to use urinals, only ever cubicles, because the risk of being seen was too daunting. This boy (who actually had nothing to worry about – then again, none of us do) had been conditioned to hate his body from everything he'd seen and heard over the years. Yet the issue wasn't his penis, it was his perspective.

Worryingly, it's a view shared by millions of men everywhere. It hides in teenage bedrooms up and down the country, regularly reinforced by pop culture of every form and calibre. Even a recent production of *King Lear* at the National Theatre featured three – yes, THREE – references to men's 'small' dicks. Integral to the plot and tastefully done? I think not. Together, this feeds a multi-million-pound juggernaut of fear, which invades every spam inbox on a daily basis with the promise of lotions, potions and perspex pumps which do more harm than good. Worse of all, it also becomes acceptable. The new normal.

When I first started writing at the *Mail*, I saw a man on *This Morning* discussing his decision to undergo a penis enlargement operation. A conversation which brought a tear to my eye (for all the right reasons). Chatting to Phillip Schofield and Holly Willoughby in a pre-recorded segment to protect his identity, the nine-minute feature peaked when before-and-after photos flashed up on screen, no doubt to cackles of laughter in the production office and across the country.

Yet, although he certainly got his money's worth, I was more amazed that this brave chap coined a phrase which nailed our obsession with size: penile dysmorphia. Borrowing terminology from body dysmorphia, which sees patients clinically preoccupied with non-existent physical faults in themselves, this bloke summed up an endemic problem with just two words. It was this – not the gory footage of the operation – which brought a tear to my eye.

See, he hadn't undergone surgery for vanity or to outdo his mates in the changing room. Why would he? None of them really care. Nor had he done it to correct a medical problem which was blighting his life (one that wouldn't have been taken seriously, even if he had). Instead, he was simply trying to undo years of taunts from women and the media which had left him psychologically scarred. The very messages which affect all males, from young boys and teenagers to war veterans. So I track down his surgeon, Dr Roberto Viel, to get an idea of what motivates his patients – and if there's a trend.

'I started doing penoplastys in 1991 after a woman asked me if we'd operate on her boyfriend, who was getting very depressed about his size,' he says from his Harley Street office, wearing day-glo scrubs. 'She'd heard about a doctor in America who did the procedure and wondered if it was available here. We investigated and, after realising it was safe, trialled it here. That was twenty-three years ago.'

Now, he says, it's their biggest seller. 'Liposuction is common and so is gynocomastia [surgery to correct 'man boobs'] but penis enlargement tops the lot. I do at least two or three cases each week. Even when the recession hit and people stopped spending money, the demand for every other procedure suffered a dip – except the penoplasty.'

Big business indeed. So, come on, how many of his patients are genuinely small? And by that I mean medically defined small. 'It's very, very rare to see a real micropenis, which affects less than 1 per cent of the male population,' he asserts.

> I've operated on a few, but the overwhelming majority of my patients have a penis that we consider average by textbook standards. Unfortunately, what we consider normal isn't necessarily what everybody else does, but it's understandable: everything tells men they're below average. It's destructive.
>
> The reality is that my patients don't come to me wanting to be porn stars, they want their lives back. They're refusing to take their sons to the swimming pool because they've focused all their anxieties and self-hate onto their penis. We consider it a psychosexual treatment. By changing a person physically we're changing them mentally. Yes, they end up with a larger penis, but ultimately they leave with a bigger sense of confidence. A better quality of life.

This all sounds very philanthropic (although the surgeries cost about £7,000 combined), but surely all this added size also improves sex, right? Not quite. 'Length isn't important,' he says. 'It all relative when combined with the size of the vagina. Increasing numbers of women are having surgeries to tighten the vaginal wall [commonly referred to as 'designer vaginas'] because they consider themselves too big, especially after childbirth.'

Which brings me to my next point. Because, if size does matter – as women often say it does – then surely it matters on them too. After all, friction is friction and their bits vary as much as ours. It reminds me of an episode from US television show *Curb Your Enthusiasm* called 'Big Vagina'. In it, the show's protagonist, Larry David, meets a nurse, Lisa, who claims she stopped dating his best friend, Jeff, because he has a small penis. When Larry later confronts him about this, it transpires it's her who has the anatomical anomaly – not him. I won't ruin the punchline, but I will say that it's better than ten years of therapy. Not least because the moral of the story is this: if she thinks you're too small, chances are it's because she's too big. After all, men can put a master key in a door, but if the lock's too big then it won't open. And that's not our fault.

A 2006 study by Barnhart, Izquierdo & Pretorius for the Kinsey Institute found the average vagina measures 62.7 mm with a relatively large range (40.8–95 mm). The position of the cervix, marking the end of the vagina, can also vary at different points in a woman's cycle, making them all shapes and sizes.

The difference between this and penis size variation? Young lads are forever told size matters, whilst girls are told they're beautiful regardless of their physical attributes. That's the irony. Women scorn the fashion industry for putting pressure on them, but – whilst I sympathise – it's these women who trash a guy because his body isn't to their liking. Even though his body is his, not theirs. Rarely is a penis respected for simply being the amazing, life-creating body part it actually is.

I was once at a friend's twenty-first birthday party, which was festooned with pictures of him at various stages in his life, including some as a child in the bath. Even here, whilst celebrating his passage into adulthood, there were women whom I overheard say: 'Hmm, he hasn't changed much … if you know what I mean.' Another time, during a man's speech about prostate cancer at a major health seminar in London, two women in the row ahead of me leaned in to each other and made an inch gesture between their thumb and forefinger. Both times, my heart sank. Not for me or my body – I'm happy – but for the death of basic manners.

Anyone would think the sole purpose of a penis was to pleasure women. Get in line, girls – they have a whole gamut of functions for their owner before anybody else even enters the room.

More importantly, the entire size debate is … well,

bollocks. Biology proves it. If male size did matter, it would affect our ability to urinate, father children and get an erection from the moment we reached puberty. Which it doesn't. Even the *Kama Sutra* explains that there are three sizes of penis and three sizes of vagina, the perfect combination of which depends on personal preference.

Instead, small is a shame we're taught about, then taunted with. Advertisers use it as a foundation on which to sell their 'remedy' products, whilst women broker it as an insecurity they alone have the power to relieve us of. Influential German psychoanalyst Karl Abraham suggested this was a vindictive form of penis envy – and, who knows, he might be right. After all, why else would people – well, let's be honest here: women – be so vile about something so amazing? If he's wrong, and he might be, then it's just simple sexism, which is worse.

Either way, it doesn't tickle. So trust me when I say that making a mental leap into healthy thinking is the cheapest, safest and most satisfying solution there is.

I once knew a guy at university who thought buying herbal growth pills from Japan would cause him to wake up with a penis like porn actor Jeff Stryker, solving all his problems. It didn't. It just cost him £45 plus import fees, one awkward trip to the Post Office and, later, embarrassing diarrhoea. He'd spend hours devising ways to pimp his penis (because of an ex's throwaway comment when he was fifteen), which essentially meant trawling websites to buy a whole manner of gadgets.

The rule of thumb was: don't ever open his post.

Thankfully, he eventually met somebody on a night out and, from that moment on, changed. Turns out the sex was mutually their best ever and, naturally, his penis was an integral part of that. Now, they're married with kids – and he's never doubted his dick since. Even though it's exactly the same as it was before.

He got off lightly, though. In recent years I've spoken with countless urologists who've seen horrifying home enlargement jobs that would cause even the toughest man to faint. There was one who used chip fat in an old glue gun to give himself bigger girth (it didn't work), another who tried to release his own suspensory ligament with a pair of kitchen scissors (don't even think about it – it didn't work) and the man who, quite literally, used Polyfilla to fill out his phallus (seriously, don't do it – it didn't work and I think he died).

Instead, we should learn from these men. They weren't home alone looking for something to do because the football season hadn't started; they were searching for solutions to their anxieties, which had completely spun out of control. OK, the above cases are extreme ones, but men everywhere are wasting hours, days, weeks and months worrying about something they can't do much about anyway. Forget worrying if your penis is short; LIFE is short.

Author and comedian Richard Herring wrote 2003's *Talking Cock* – the male equivalent to *The Vagina Monologues*. In it he noted that men's paranoia about their size is so deeply ingrained (and encouraged) by society that we don't even question it:

> Few of us are going to be prepared to rock the boat and look at the positive things that men do – to focus on all the men who are being good fathers, good lovers, good friends … for fear of appearing un-manly … Rather than making the obvious mental leap and concluding that the male stereotype was wrong, I had decided there was something wrong with me.

One easy, immediate and fun way to do this is by viewing porn with reality glasses. Not literally, of course, but by simply understanding that the actors in them are no more atypical than the pneumatic blondes they're with.

'I was always careful to point out the actual rarity of penises over 8 inches,' says publishing editor Dian Hanson, referring to her work on Taschen's *The Big Penis Book*. 'Seriously, I can't tell you how many thousands of photographs I had to examine to find ones of that size.'

Interestingly, proportionate to body scale, man already

has the biggest penis of all the primates – but does bigger always mean better? I enter the online world of Craigslist to find out. In the personals section I find a man who's advertising his 11-inch penis to women with pride, which thus begins a very unusual email exchange. When he eventually agrees to speak with me, he admits that he frequently fails to get it completely up because a bigger dick requires so much more blood flow than normal. Even then, its heaviness means it often fails to stand at the optimum erect angle. Still envious? Thought not.

In 2012, a man called Patrick Moote learned self-acceptance the hard way. He got down on one knee and proposed to his then girlfriend at a UCLA basketball game in Los Angeles. Crushingly, before an audience of thousands, she said no – later telling Moote that it was because his penis wasn't big enough. Gutted, he became an overnight phenomenon when the clip of her rejection went viral, being watched more than 10 million times in four days.

Already on the world stage, penis in hand, he pragmatically decided to answer the size question in a documentary – or is it cockumentary? – called *UnHung Hero*. According to the film, which was endorsed by *Fahrenheit 9/11* director Michael Moore, the US penis size industry is worth a whopping $5 billion. Gentlemen, that's $5 BILLION WORTH OF SELF-LOATHING

AND SHAME which could be spent on so many better things. Specifically, things that work. DO NOT GIVE IT ANY MORE.

'The fear comes from the fact that we've all been led to believe what's "average" is huge, when, in reality, most of us are walking around within an inch of one another. Yet, whenever it's talked about it's always in extremes – "so small" or "so big!" – when, even across cultures, the difference in size is not as drastic as most people think,' he tells me.

> Besides, being insecure about having a small penis is way worse then actually having a small penis. The average female vagina is only 3.5 inches deep, and the clitoris is right up front, so it doesn't matter anyway. The best thing guys can do is become informed. The film taught me that confidence is the cure for just about anything. If you are owning it then no one else will even care.

One man who knows this all too well was British film-maker Lawrence Barraclough. Armed with a penis that's 3.5 inches erect, he spent years agonising over his size until he finally faced his issues in a BBC Three documentary called *My Penis and I*. Groundbreaking for British television, it rugby-tackled women's fascism with size and translated it into something positive for the guys.

Once again, Barraclough's issues weren't innate or justified – they were simply acquired from a toxic narrative in the wider world. 'My penis insecurities stemmed from being laughed at by everybody who came into contact with my dick,' he told me. 'Right from my first sexual experience.'

In a bid to be accepted, he considered everything from completely avoiding sexual relationships to surgery, which either sees fat transferred from love handles and pumped into the shaft, or erection ligaments slashed so it hangs lower when flaccid (although only when flaccid – in fact, this tactic can give men 'dive-bomber dicks' that hang down, even when erect).

'It stopped being an option for me when I was told how little I'd gain and how potentially dangerous it could be,' he added.

> I tried a penis pump a few times but I just found the whole thing a little too dispiriting. Ultimately, what set me free from my size concerns was being open and talking about them. When the film aired I thought people would see my penis and laugh at me all over again, but that couldn't have been further from the truth. Since making *My Penis and I*, not one person has said anything derogatory about my cock. Instead, they congratulate me on sharing such a personal story so publicly. I'm also

a father now, which my penis had a small part in, so I couldn't possibly be anything other than happy with it. My penis made that happen. It's pretty amazing.

Abso-fucking-lutely. So can we definitively say, once and for all, that size doesn't matter?

'Yes, definitely,' says leading psychosexual therapist Phillip Hodson.

We live in a bigness culture where most women know that many male insecurities are penis-focused, so belittling their endowment is a power-play. Fortunately, there's no penis that is too small to give some pleasure – even if it's just a 'bud' then it's still as hot as the external part of a woman's clitoris.

Besides, when it comes to experience, does not possessing a 10-inch penis really stop you having the fuck of your life? Answers on a postcard, please...

Author Susie Orbach once said that fat was a feminist issue. If that's true, then penis size is an issue of the same scale for men. Now, thanks to the likes of Lawrence Barraclough, Larry David and Patrick Moote, millions of men might just stand an inch or two taller because they appreciate the politics of the penis.

So, the next time you're about to sleep with somebody

who looks at your dick and asks 'Who's that going to please?' the only answer should be: 'Me.' Not only does this ensure you're the custodian of your own dick dignity, but it proves you've got the balls to tackle size sexism head on.

Now that's big.

LADS' MAGS:
A STORM IN A D-CUP

WHEN POMPEII WAS EXCAVATED BY the Victorians in the 1860s, they found a stash of porn belonging to the Romans – which, to 'protect' society, they swiftly hid in a mausoleum of smut we now know as the Secret Museum in Naples.

Jump forward 150 years and history is repeating itself with the same moral panic. Except, rather than an archaeological dig, male sexuality is now suffering a snide dig at the hands of self-appointed censors with *Downton Abbey* ideals.

So, when *Nuts* folded in April 2014, it wasn't just the end of a magazine – it was also the demise of another everyday freedom: the ability to legally enjoy human sexuality without shame. You know, the stuff we take for granted in a post-sexual revolution society.

And, according to experts, it's only going to get worse.

During its decade-long run, the glossy title may not have been the epitome of good taste, but it certainly had a place in the market, with no shortage of fans. So why did it close? Well, all it started when far-left groups demanded censorship rather than centrefolds, and in latter years, the campaigners at Lose the Lads' Mags associated it with domestic violence and misogynistic men. Although unfounded, these claims weren't good PR, and – combined with an industry-wide drop in print sales – the beginning of the end was swift in coming.

In a bid to have it banned from supermarket shelves, along with *FHM* and *Zoo*, the hard-line campaigners at the helm, UK Feminista and OBJECT, used equality legislation to scare retailers into submission, threatening legal action if they continued as stockists. The crucial point, they said – at a stretch – was that expecting staff members to sell such material was tantamount to sexual harassment and could result in expensive pay-offs.

The magazine's publisher, IPC Inspire, eloquently hit back, describing the attack as 'an unreasonable attempt to prevent shoppers from freely browsing a magazine that's already displayed according to Home Office guidelines'. Managing Director Paul Williams added:

> The objection that niche lobby groups have against certain sectors of the media should not mean that the right to purchase a perfectly legal product is restricted for the over half a million readers. This is no longer a question of whether you like men's magazines, it's a question of how far you can restrict the public's ability to consume free and legal media before it becomes censorship.

It was a very modern battle of the sexes, if not a bun fight.

Opponents presented cleverly spun statistics from self-esteem studies, but there was no robust, reliable proof of direct, scientific cause and effect. Not even close. In fact, according to the British Crime Survey, the opposite is true: when lads' mags first debuted in the mid-1990s, shifting millions of copies each month, incidents of domestic violence actually fell by 64 per cent between 1997 and 2009, whilst the number of sexual assault victims also decreased between 2004 and 2008: a statistic that directly correlates with sales.

Similar accusations that they caused children to become 'sexualised' also fell flat. Reg Bailey, chief executive of the Mothers' Union, led an independent review into this alleged side effect, hoping to find some justification for all the bluster, but awkwardly noted on page 80 of his report that, actually, 'there is no clear evidence of a causal link' between sexualised images on lads' mags and 'harm to young people'.

It was an embarrassment. It was also solid proof that societies can recede as well as progress. Just look at 1930s Berlin – indulgent partying one minute, intolerance the next. Yet, somehow, all the hysteria stuck. One high-street retailer demanded *Nuts* begin using shame-inducing 'modesty bags' – typically seen with XXX hardcore porn rags – or face being dumped altogether. The editors defiantly refused – and ultimately went, er, bust.

Yet, undeterred, the genre lives on. *Loaded* magazine, the original men's monthly, famous for its bold journalism and subsequent ladette movement, is now enjoying a major revival, whilst the remaining lads' mags are busy evolving, increasingly shape-shifting into digital formats, where demand remains consistently high.

Then again, we shouldn't be surprised by this: the

desire for erotica has always existed. Statues of a topless Venus, the goddess of love, pre-date civilisation and are considered the earliest examples of figuritive art, whilst one world-famous artefact from Egypt, the Turin Erotic Papyrus, is dubbed the lads' mag of its day (1150 BC, to be precise) by archaeologists for its raunchy depictions of nudity. You can forget E. L. James, too. John Cleland's book *Fanny Hill* doesn't just have a comedy name – it's considered the world's breakthrough in graphic literature. Originally published in 1748, it sparked the first case of US censorship thanks to its tales of BDSM and anal, which – nearly 300 years ago – was long before our parents were thumbing *Lady Chatterley's Lover* in the conservatory.

'There have been so many attempts at preventing sexual material, but, for the most part, it's uncontrollable,' says Julie Peakman, author of *The Pleasure's All Mine: A History of Perverse Sex*. 'You only need to look at how porn has, at least in part, led the development of technology. It existed in print back in the Renaissance period, in cinemas in the early twentieth century, and now on the internet.'

Still, the drive to control it remains strong – which might explain why Britain is, perhaps surprisingly, one of the most censored countries in the European Union.

'Hardcore porn has only been available here since

2000 – and that only happened because it was already on the internet,' says Jerry Barnett, founder of campaign group Sex and Censorship who challenge porn scaremongering.

To this day it has never been allowed on British TV and we're just one of three EU countries who do this. The US has hardcore porn and twenty-five other European member states allow it, but here even subscribe channels like Television X can't show penetration of any kind. If they accidentally load the explicit European tape in the UK player they'll get a fine of £25,000 from Ofcom. It's very punitive.

What most men fail to realise is that we have a state machine that's dedicated to stopping people viewing porn – and, if we're not careful, we're about to see the same applied to the internet. We're about to lose the freedom we've had online for twenty-five years.

On the one hand there are bodies like Ofcom and the Department for Culture, Media and Sport who randomly censor on our behalf – then, on the other hand, there's the morality campaigners who create panic and conditions for censorship to take place. Until the turn of the century many of these were Christians or religious fuddy-duddies like Mary Whitehouse, but Britain has become much less religious, so these arguments don't work anymore. The rise

of feminist morality has replaced it – but there's very little difference between the two groups: they use the same
tactics and the same kinds of language.

According to him, the next big crackdown is mobile
phone content.

'We also have very repressive content possession laws.
To restrict what can be distributed is one thing, but to
restrict what people possess is another – it means you can
have something sent to you in a WhatsApp message and
you become a sex offender.'

To flesh this out I approach an expert. 'Let me tell you
a legal joke,' says leading obscenity lawyer Myles Jackman.

> A man walks into a court. He's charged with an offence
> under Section 63 of the Criminal Justice and Immi-
> gration Act 2008 of being in possession of an 'extreme
> pornographic' video of a woman having sex with a tiger.
>
> The video was sent to him by a friend, unsolicited,
> as a joke. He had no idea what the content of the video
> was before opening it. Yet the defendant was arrested
> at his home address, interviewed by the police under
> caution, charged, then bailed to the Magistrates' Court
> and finally sent to the Crown Court. It was here that
> the judge requested the video be played in full, with the
> sound on, in open court.

The play button was pressed.

It turned out the 'tiger' was a man in a tiger-skin costume, who turns to the camera and says: 'That's grrrreat!' Hilarious. Except that the joke was on the defendant, Andrew Holland, of Wrexham, north Wales, as the story was on the front cover of the *Daily Telegraph* and in numerous articles published across the globe. His name became synonymous with the joke, which had a devastating impact on his reputation.

The Crown Prosecution Service are now reviewing the law.

But what is everybody so afraid of? Porn barely even has a rebellious streak anymore. What was once subversive and exciting (why was it always in bushes and broken shop windows?) is now turning academic, with scholarly publishers Routledge printing the new, official *Porn Studies* journal. Like Hugh Hefner guest-editing *The Lancet*, it's 'the first dedicated, international, peer-reviewed journal to critically explore those cultural products and services designated as pornographic and their economic, historical, institutional, legal and social contexts'. Blimey.

Specifically, one of their key findings is that at least 30 per cent of online porn users are women, which helps destroy the myth that it is simply sexist.

The people behind it, university professors Clarissa

Smith and Feona Attwood – women! – studied more than 5,000 people on their sex-viewing trends. Among their findings they also found that men's use of visual material can't simply be dismissed as an aggressive, one-way exercise of projecting their hardcore fantasies onto wipe-clean pages. In fact, the opposite is true. It reaffirmed something we, as men, have always known: that it's more multi-faceted than that. *We* are more multi-faceted than that.

Aside from feeling horny, which is an obvious incentive, men view porn for a variety of valid reasons: to get in the mood (with, or for, their partner), to reconnect with their body or, sometimes, just because they simply can't sleep (oh, come on, we've all been there!). Additionally, hundreds said they viewed porn because they were inquisitive about acts they'd consider doing in the future, which means they were exploring their desires in a safe, consequence-free way – something *Nuts* was part of.

'At their height, lads' mags offered men a space in which to consider their bodies, relationships and identities in ways that weren't really available anywhere else,' says Jude Roberts of Birkbeck College.

> Traditional ideas about masculinity don't allow much
> space for consideration of men's anxieties about their
> bodies, their sex lives or their relationships, so whilst
> lads' mags are far from a bastion of progressive gender

politics, they do provide their readers with a more complex view of masculinity than many other types of media.

Agreed. So, hang on – if we know there's no proven link
between men accessing porn and society's evils – what
exactly is the problem? Why can women go into a shop
like Ann Summers and buy a dildo or read clit-lit, yet men
are restricted in buying a legally permissible magazine in
which models pose freely. Have I missed something? Am
I going mad? Or can somebody please name and claim
the 7-tonne elephant in the room?

'When I was in my early twenties, *Loaded* magazine
came onto the market and scared the shit out of me. I
knew nothing of human sexuality. I'd had sex, but not
explored who I was as a sexual being. And, it goes without saying, I knew even less about male sexuality. So I
was confused,' says Paula Wright, an academic who, in
her spare time, performs a stand-up comedy smackdown
on the idea that sexy isn't sexist. Yep, the radical notion
that men finding women attractive isn't discrimination.

The feminist rhetoric at the time fuelled that fear. Men
were out to get us, to humiliate us. But it was just another
salvo response across the barricades. The truth is that it's
all about power. The urge to control female sexuality is
about keeping their exchange rate with men high.

She points me in the direction of a study called 'Cultural Suppression of Female Sexuality' by Florida University professors Roy Baumeister and Jean Twenge. It states: 'Sex is a resource that men desire and women possess. To obtain sex, men must offer women other desired resources in return, such as money, commitment, security, attention or respect.' In other words, life's a marketplace where women are the sellers and men are the buyers. Like eBay, but played out in restaurants and nightclubs.

'The harder it is for men to obtain sex, the more they'll be willing to offer women in return,' it continues.

> Sexual scarcity improves women's bargaining position … whilst the general suppression of female sexuality reduces the risk that each woman will lose her male lover to another woman. Throughout history men have been willing to leave one woman for another, especially when the new one is sexually more appealing.

Explosive? Yes, but also true. It's the classic 'treat them mean, keep them keen' incentive – which is undermined when the lads' mags give it away. Trouble is, the internet has already thwarted this. Sex is already out there.

More importantly, who exactly do these objectors represent? Is their campaign the result of a lengthy consultation with the glamour models themselves – women

who, terrified of their readership, ran to them for help?
Is this actually some makeshift workers' union – or just a
storm in a D-cup? 'They haven't spoken to me or any of
the women I know, so they certainly don't represent us,'
says Hayley Ann Newnes, a model who's appeared in *Zoo*,
FHM and *Nuts*. 'Nobody bothered to ask us for our opinions. They assume either we're too stupid to understand
or will contradict them. It's classic propaganda. They're
the ones using us for their own gratification, not men.'

I put this to both UK Feminista and OBJECT, but
am greeted with radio silence. Lose the Lads' Mags have
suddenly lost their voice.

'I grew up in a family with a lot of feminists and,
although they might not like my career path, they ultimately respect it,' Newnes tells me.

> The old feminism used choice as their mantra – that
> summed up the movement in the '60s and '70s: choice
> to have an abortion; choice to sleep with whoever you
> want; choice to use contraception. Now, modern femi-
> nists focus on buzzwords such as 'objectification', which
> might sound good, but actually just hide the fact they're
> attacking other peoples' choices. There's no logic behind
> it. It's simply women attacking other women.
>
> Quite frankly, if feminism is about making choices,
> why are feminists the only ones trying to take choice

away from me? I'm not brainwashed – this is a decision I made.

Plus, I've always been treated with respect on shoots. Many of them are women-led too. I've had several jobs with female photographers and female-dominated crews. This is a very big part of what objectors choose to ignore because it weakens their case. It's not a black-and-white issue of one gender versus another – there are women who photograph, market, manage, produce, edit and promote these products. There's no oppressive force making them do this, it's their career. They're knowingly, happily making money from it.

To get a greater sense of this reality, I catch up with Martin Daubney, former editor of *Loaded* magazine and now a journalist at Sky News and *The Sun*. We meet at the Royal Institute of British Architects, just around the corner from the BBC's Broadcasting House – where, co-incidentally, he's just been cross-examined on air as part of *Woman's Hour*, which – in the 200-yard dash to meet me – has evolved into Twitter trolling. Nice. Thankfully, a quick drink and he's back on form, happy to chat about the halcyon days and the 'good place' it all came from.

'A lot of people don't believe me, but we were all attracted to *Loaded* for its gonzo journalism and live-for-today attitude, rather than the women,' he tells me.

I was always accused of being sexist for not having more women on the team, but there weren't many men on *Marie Claire* either. *Loaded* was born into a vacuum of men being told how to behave. Back then it was all about the New Man, the north London-living, touchy-feely man who wasn't afraid to cry. The type of man who surrendered his masculinity to fit into a new world order. *Loaded* was a two-fingered gesture to men becoming more asexual.

A father of two, Daubney is an articulate and considered force, not to mention an ideal ambassador for the genre. Anything but the Neanderthal his haters might expect, he's actually a cool, calm, everyman figure – even in the epicentre of an online assault which sees his phone ping with updates of endless, unwelcome alerts.

Back then it was desperately unfashionable to fight, drink and take drugs – even just to be a man – but then Oasis and the Happy Mondays emerged. Suddenly, footie fans who used to beat each other up would be hugging on dance floors. Ecstasy and music brought men together, but so did lads' mags. Of course, the liberal media said we should be at home doing domestic chores and raising children full-time, but *Loaded* rejected all that – and represented how men felt. It was a private club – or it certainly felt like that back in the day. It was a space to be male without apology, where it was acceptable to be a bloke. It even celebrated the downsides – flatulence, getting drunk, being unfaithful and getting VD. It accepted that men were flawed and didn't patronise them for it. At the same time, it also didn't listen to all the criticisms, of which there were many.

Specifically, *Loaded* was even debated in Parliament, but the more readers got called sexist and reprobate, the more it reinforced their view that what they were buying was valid. Intolerance pushed men into the arms of it all. It was that Millwall attitude of: 'If you don't like it, we don't care. In fact, we like the fact you hate us, so fuck off.'

Originally, he tells me, women weren't the main shop window of the store. In the beginning, it was all about us guys.

Scan through old issues and you'll see that all the biggest football, movie and rock stars were speaking with us. Men like Jerry Springer and Michael Caine were on the cover, not women. Sure, they were part of it too, but they weren't the main part. They featured more as retro glamour models from the '80s, reinvented for bits of acceptable titillation between ground-breaking, quality journalism.

The big change only came later, thanks to Liz Hurley. She fronted an issue the same week she wore *that* infamous Versace safety-pin dress at the *Four Weddings and a Funeral* premiere with Hugh Grant, sending sales stratospheric.

> That success created pressure from upstairs. We needed more women, so the next change was our Readers' Girlfriends feature; a take on Readers' Wives, but without the net curtains and women who looked like Steve Davis. This tapped into the girl-next-door community, which men loved because they were real. It was very British and very celebratory, but also of an era where women were totally and utterly complicit. Then, the girls on the telly got involved. Donna Air, Kelly Brook and Sara Cox all used this enormous media platform to further their careers.

Which is precisely where the objectification argument fails. If you look at it commercially, it's men – not women – who are (quite happily) being 'taken advantage of' in the lads' mag exchange. Look at it like a business model, rather than a glamour model, for a moment: these titles are a device by publishers to make money. To do this they get journalists and creatives to sit in a room and think of ways to convince a particular audience – in this case, men – to part with their money in exchange for some nice pictures of attractive women and a few sparse, auxiliary words such as 'Cor!' or 'Fit!'. The models themselves get paid a wheelbarrow full of cash, whilst female celebs ride the coat tails of its success.

It's the mag buyers who are out of pocket, nervously picking the damn thing up off the shelves, looking at it waiting for something to happen. With every turn of a page they are subtly, very cleverly, being manipulated by marketeers. And they know this. They're in on it too, which is why it's a fair transaction. Nobody is being ripped off. On the contrary, people are making a fortune – from us. Which begs the question: shouldn't men be calling for a brand of men's magazine that addresses real men's issues, alongside the joy of sex, rather than something that takes their money and fobs them off with a few pictures they can get for free on the internet? PEOPLE AT THE TOP, GET ON IT.

FHM was making £17 million annual profit for EMAP, which was as much as the rest of the business combined. Everybody in the media looked at it as the template for success. Then, the weekly titles like *Zoo* and *Nuts* came in and commercially finessed the offering. The outside world will always think it was made by pornographers, but actually the opposite is true. It was produced by

some of the most highly skilled magazine brains ever. It
was owned by Time Warner: the biggest magazine cor-
poration in the world.

Interestingly, *Nuts* didn't start off as a controversy –
initially it was a relatively tame title, which failed to
connect with its market.

People later accused it of dumbing down, but – despite
being bankrolled by £6 million – the original launch
[owned by the man who now runs *Shortlist* magazine]
was taken to market research after seven weeks because
it wasn't working. Guess what the feedback was? More
women.

It's an over-simplification to say the men's market is
just a load of cavemen or perverts. *Loaded* was a real-
time exercise in product-finessing. Yes, it was a magazine
produced by 100 people in a slightly haphazard way, but
we also reported to shareholders in the world's biggest
media conglomerate. We were the bastard child who did
well. Ask any man from the team what his favourite bit
of the job was and none of them will say the girls – it
was always the creative, journalistic side.

Indeed. But when I ask if he's ever tried explaining this
to Kat Banyard, the campaign director for Lose the Lads'

Mags, it appears Israel and Palestine might have a better chance of peace talks. 'I've debated with her several times but it goes in one ear and out the other,' he says. 'I've asked for solid proof that lads' mags cause harm, but she can't present it – because it doesn't exist. Then again, they use the same lawyer who defends serial killer Ian Brady, which says it all.'

So what exactly is their motivation? What's in it for them?

'It's all about money and control – of which there's a wealth of both in censorship,' adds Jerry Barnett.

> The BBFC [which puts age certificates on films] was a voluntary body until 1984. Then, they created the moral panic around video nasties – and got statutory power to make selling videos without a BBFC rating illegal. Last year they turned over something like £6 million, so persuading the government to give you a monopoly is a nice little earner. They're a business.
>
> OBJECT are very good at creating one campaign after another, which is all designed to give the impression that things are getting worse. Why? Because there's money in it. They already have several full-time employees, so it's clearly not doing too badly. And don't forget there are grants for groups who call themselves women's human rights organisations.

When I submit a freedom of information request to OBJECT, asking for details of how much they get – if anything – in grants and how many paying members they have, they once again fail to respond. But, then again, they don't really need to: on their site they encourage people to become paid members, stating: 'Membership is one of our key sources of income and every member's contribution makes a difference: just ten members can bring £600 of income per year, every year, meaning that we can continue to plan and run our groundbreaking campaigns in the future.'

Suddenly, it all becomes clear. These people won't mind their own business because it *is* their business. Literally.

That said, this doesn't mean similar arguments against page three, for example, aren't sound – do we really need naked breasts in a national newspaper? The last time I checked, cleavage hadn't affected the national debt or affected UN relations. It's in the wrong context. But, at the same time, allowing men to autonomously enjoy lads' mags is not a luxury to be grateful for. We do not need permission to consume something legal. Women do not own sex.

People forget this. They also forget that men enjoy these publications on a much wider spectrum of content alongside newspapers, biographies, sports pages, text books and style mags. Erotic pictures are also not the only representation of women they'll ever see. They will have real-time interactions with them in their families, workplaces and circle of friends, where I'm assuming the women don't spend every hour on the point of orgasm in a sultry pose. Well, unless they know Helen Flanagan, of course.

This is because these men, like all men, have rounded lives, which is why it's so utterly patronising to say they can't appreciate adult content for what it is – something sexual, in a moment, to meet or enhance a need.

To our credit, most of us already know this – even if the messages we receive about it are, at best, contradictory and, at worst, unfair. See, whilst one side are trying to ban boobs, others are trying to liberate them. Across the Atlantic there's a campaign called Free the Nipple, which – as the name suggests – is asking the world's media to stop pixelating women's breasts because, in doing so, they're censoring them. This, they claim, keeps women in a perpetual loop of cultural repression. Cara Delevingne, Liv Tyler and Rumer Willis are already supporters.

To learn more I speak with Lina Esco, the 29-year-old rudder steering the movement from LA. She tells me it's still illegal for a woman to be topless in thirty-seven US states – even if they're breast-feeding – and, before I know it, we're bonding over mammary glands. Bosom buddies, indeed. Who'd have thought it?

'What America needs is a full blast of boobies every-where until everybody just calms down,' she jokes. 'In Louisiana you can get three years in prison for getting them out – it's insane, no?'

I agree, but – apparently – many others don't. In particular, the response from women has been a mixed bag, she admits. 'We've had some really great support and some real hate, but we're trying to educate them. It's like John Lennon said: don't hate what you don't understand.'

Sounds like something we can relate to. Then again, if she's encouraging toplessness in cities around the world, doesn't she worry about men constantly 'perving' on them when they're shopping at Walmart or on the school run?

> No, not at all – you can't change the way men see boobs and we wouldn't want to. If they view it as a sexual thing, great, that's up to them. Naturally, just because boobs are out doesn't mean they can be touched, but men already know this. In fact, men first fought for the right to go topless in the early 1900s, so we're just following your lead.

'Really?' I say, surprised.

> Yeah. It was illegal for men to be topless in the US for a long time. They had to wear one-piece suits constantly,

even in the summer. Thousands of them were getting arrested because they refused to comply. It wasn't until 1934 when four men from Coney Island fought back with topless protests and changed the legislation, so actually you guys did it first.

See, I told you we were brilliant.

But what about all this fuss with our lads' mags then?

Live and let live, that's what I say. If men want something that turns them on and the models want to pose for them, that's their choice – there's no reason for anybody to shut them down. Women enjoy *Cosmopolitan*, men enjoy *FHM*. That's the way we are. If people don't like it, read something else – or start another magazine with a different approach, but don't censor. We need to protect freedom of expression and freedom of press.

This is something British journalist Lulu Le Vay agrees with. She started out as deputy editor of fanzine *Sleazenation* in the mid-1990s, later becoming a music and lifestyle writer for *The Face*, *i-D*, *The Independent* and *The Observer*. She was also a militant feminist who loathed lads' mags with a passion – that is, until she worked on one and wrote about the experience for major left-wing title the *New Statesman*.

'I never thought I'd be the one who ended up defending these types of magazines,' she tells me.

> I really detested them and was very judgemental about the men reading them. But, after working on one, I realised how much young women desperately wanted to be featured in them and how the men there were extremely respectful. Similarly, the copy was never sexual or derogatory, and there was a great deal of other content aside from girls, such as TV, music, games, sports – all the stuff young men like to read about. This subject matter was approached in the same professional way if it were a car or music magazine. It forced me to think about it in a different way – and it did break down some of my stuffy and judgemental barriers. Not just regarding the type of men who'd be working on them, but the girls modelling and the readers too.

Unsurprisingly, when she shared this experience, Lulu realised the unpalatable, ironic truth that – actually – it was other women, not men, who were the ones being sexist.

> The response from women was not good. I even had to block one person from my Facebook page because she was bombarding me with angry messages. but,

fortunately, that's not all women. Interestingly, my PhD supervisor, who is a well-known feminist academic, introduced me to a body of work exploring similar issues in the US, whilst there were also a few women who contacted me directly to say they found my angle refreshing.

I'm not an advocate for lads' magazines, but ultimately it's about the constant battle women have with the right to do what they want with their bodies.

When she puts it like this, it's a no-brainer.

When I was a boy, my mother was a counsellor at an abortion clinic in Liverpool. I'd often go there in the school holidays and play in the empty waiting room. One day, as we arrived on a seemingly normal morning, the street was crammed with people. Loud pro-life people, mostly women – I might add – with banners. As we approached the bright red front door of the BPAS building, the crowd jeered, spat and pushed – even at me, a child.

These self-appointed freedom fighters – fiercely claiming to represent the moral future, the way forward, the majority – thought they were civil rights heroes, but actually, they failed to recognise that they were more like the new oppressives. Why? *Because the people they were claiming to liberate were already free.*

As we jostled through them – placards waving, whistles

blowing, my dad trying to shield us – he explained very calmly and in hushed tones that, sometimes, people are so passionate about a cause, so indoctrinated by their version of truth, so desperate for it to survive and thrive, that nothing is off limits – and, sometimes, they become exactly what they claim to oppose.

Years later, whilst writing this chapter, I remember these words – and look them up. Turns out famous philosopher Friedrich Nietzsche said something similar: 'Beware that, when fighting "monsters", you yourself do not become a monster. For when you gaze long into the abyss, the abyss also gazes into you.'

Somebody might want to tell Lose the Lads' Mags this. Because whenever I see them in action, I remember these words, see the weakness in their extremism and cringe.

SEX ISN'T SEXIST

AT THE RISK OF QUOTING '90s hip-hop trio Salt-N-Pepa, let's talk about sex. Not just because it's one of life's greatest pleasures – well, unless you're Max Mosley, poor guy – but because none of us would be here without it.

Whatever you call it – intercourse, making love, fucking, schtupping, boning, bumming … oh no, not bumming – sex made us. Sex is what stops civilisation from coughing and wheezing its way into oblivion. It is, almost literally, the Big Bang of human existence. A biological masterstroke. The circle of life's pivotal starting point (by which I mean the cradle-to-grave metaphor – not Elton John's song of the same name, obviously).

Essentially, we owe it all to sex.

So it's surprising, and perhaps a little ungrateful, that it's long been given a bum deal – and not in a good way. First it ended up on the cutting-room floor when the Virgin Mary conceived baby Jesus, then religious finger-waggers branded it sinful until the swinging '60s – but, even then, legislation kept it on a tight leash without the slightest hint of adventurous role-play.

Thankfully, these days, we are much more relaxed. Channel 4 has already had real-life couples shagging on live TV, branches of Agent Provocateur line the high street, vibrators are bought like toasters and the biggest literary hit of recent years is *Fifty Shades of Grey* – a book consumed by women of all ages, in all places, at all times of the day and night, from busy trains on the morning commute to Kindles in care homes. Its sado-masochistic subject matter is no longer an extreme fetish to be gasped at, pearls clutched, but the title of a Rihanna track played at family weddings.

Female sexuality has never been such a casual, and comfortable, cultural reference point.

So it's bizarre that whilst public attitudes around women's desires have relaxed, those concerning men's have, well, stiffened. Not just in relation to how we consume erotica in public, with tacky 'titty bars' and the like being frowned upon – that's nothing new – but privately, in our homes, and increasingly, our minds.

Men enjoying sex has become sexist.

American journalist Tom Junod experienced this first-hand when he published an op-ed piece in *Esquire* noting the appeal of 42-year-old women. Sure, he may have a career that includes two of the industry's most prestigious accolades, plus acclaim for his landmark piece identifying 9/11's 'falling man', but even that didn't exempt him from a good old-fashioned bollocking. In fact, he was publicly savaged by critics who said he had no right to voice an opinion – even though what he wrote was, er, an opinion piece.

Columnists everywhere from Jezebel to the BBC queued up to say he was reprehensible for such 'offensive' beliefs, presumably because, in their eyes, it was default discrimination against every woman who wasn't yet forty-two, or who had been but wasn't anymore. The scale of response was so exaggerated that the *LA Times* assigned five writers to it, whilst Gawker reported the story three times.

'They said I declared 42-year-olds fuckable, which isn't true,' he tells me during a transatlantic call when the dust finally settles, six weeks later. 'But the facts soon became irrelevant – it quickly morphed into something else, something aggressive and personal, which is a shame because I wrote it honourably.'

So what happened?

> Well, we had Cameron Diaz on the cover and, because she's forty-two, we wanted to write about her with a fresh, positive angle. Naturally, because *Esquire*'s ethos is the public admiration of women, it absolutely came from a good place, but amid the madness it was almost deliberately misinterpreted in sinister ways.

Five days of online trolling and personal attacks followed, along with calls for an editorial retraction. The vehemence, even violence, with which people expressed themselves was alarming. One hater said, 'I just looked you up on Wikipedia and I see that you're fifty-five. Oh, yeah! That is such a hot age. It's like, you're still alive, but only for about thirty more years,' whilst another chimed in: 'We're going to beat down that sad man's door…'

Christ, he might've had a better time criticising the Prophet Muhammed in the Middle East.

> When it exploded I spoke to my editor and he told me: 'Tom, the good news is it'll only last thirty-six hours. The bad news is you're only in hour one,' but, actually, it

went on for nearly a week. It became hypnotic. Almost medieval. I felt like I was witnessing a different side of human behaviour. People were declaring me old and dried up. That I couldn't get laid. That I was a pervert and a creep. My age was a pivotal part of the attack, too. They said I had saggy balls and that my dick was never gonna be used again. For all their protestations about ageism, they themselves became ageist.

But did they at least have a point?

No! Look, I understand that some men are assholes and of course it's fine for people to say the article was badly written or whatever, that's cool. But there's absolutely nothing noble in what they did. I have a wife, she's fifty-six, and we have a daughter – yet I was treated like a serial misogynist. The culmination of the insanity was when Rebecca Traister at the *New Republic* likened my views to the women of the Hobby Lobby being denied contraception by the Supreme Court. It was madness. At one point the overreaction was so severe I considered leaving Twitter, but I thought: why the hell should I? I'm not being chased away by the mob. That's just censorious.

Amid the shrilling, the message – although never explicitly stated – was clear: 'good' men will diplomatically find all women equally attractive, all the time, forever – which I can only assume is like giving every child a prize in a party game.

Then again, when Alex Bilmes, UK editor of *Esquire*, said the role of all its female models (across all adult ages!) was somewhat 'ornamental', at least for its readers in that specific instance, he too kicked up a storm. Speaking at a conference on feminism in the media, he made the startling revelation that the monthly glossy is – shock, horror – a men's magazine. He earnestly said:

> We produce a title that has a male gaze, and this is the controversial bit that people don't like, but I always tell the truth about it – the women we feature in the magazine are ornamental, that is how we see them. Heterosexual men regard women in many ways, as their wife, sister, daughter or mother … but there are certain times we just want to look at them because they're sexy. [In that instance] they are there to be a beautiful object, like a cool car.

You know, the same way *Heat* and *Marie Claire* feature naked men.

Yet, sure enough, he was publicly lambasted, with one website naming him 'Douche of the Day' and *The Guardian* – of course – asking if he'd 'escaped from a *Benny Hill* sketch'.

Hilariously, all this self-righteous fury erupted after decades of women portraying men on a binary scale of either a) boring in bed/unable to make women orgasm/incapable of finding a clitoris/emotionally retarded/lacking endurance or b) creepy, predatory and perverse.

In Hadley Freeman's *Be Awesome*, for example, she says men who like women with Brazilian bikini waxes are – and I quote – 'lazy, selfish jerks or paedophiles', which is perhaps slightly over-thinking the style of a person's pubic hair. But, let's run with it anyway, because surely this also means a woman's corresponding preference about, I don't know, a man's hairy shoulders or his smooth 'back, sack and crack' equates to the same thing.

Ah, no – of course not, because that would be a cougar! And they're ace! Let's make a film about them! We'll call it *Notes on a Scandal*! Judi Dench will do it! It won't be the story of a woman who cheats on her husband to shag a minor, oh no. Instead, it will be a cerebral, artistic, empowering examination of the deep-seated sexual and emotional rapids that run at the heart of every woman, whilst the men are off being dirty pervs in raincoats. Give me a fucking break.

Firstly, let's get something straight: a twenty-year-old woman with shaved pubic hair looks like a twenty-year-old woman with shaved pubic hair, *not* a child. Secondly, women do not dictate what men find attractive.

Blimey, it's no wonder we're all retreating into commercialised sex, where the customer is always right – or at least always *feels* right. There's less risk of repercussion in a pay-per-view person. Then again, even this is under fire. Five years ago the government pushed through the Policing and Crime Bill 2009, which gave local councils across Britain the power to shut law-abiding strip bars at random. The latest is Spearmint Rhino in central London. Yep, Richard Branson may be on the verge of selling tickets to the moon and sperm can be bought online, but free-thinking adults can't pay somebody to dance in an over-priced bit of cotton-blend. Go figure.

Tellingly, supporters of these moral-compass clampdowns do nothing – at all, ever – to close gay sex clubs. And nor should they. But it does make me wonder: why the disparity? Why are gay men more entrusted with testosterone than their straight brothers? Is it because, if they went feral and suddenly attacked someone, their victim would be male, not female? Wow. I'm sure Peter Tatchell would be delighted with that.

Either way, men's enjoyment of sex is the new, low-hanging fruit for our biggest critics – and, at its core, is shame. But how the hell did we end up here? Weren't we all supposed to be liberated and new age about this by now?

'When I was in college during the mid-1960s, heady

dreams of liberation filled the air. Hippies were practising free love whilst European art films embodied a sophisticated model of sexual expression,' says Camille Paglia, tell-it-like-it-is author, professor and feminist talking head who, funnily enough, happily discusses *giving* head – albeit not personally, but professionally, as an expert on sexual politics.

> The high point of that period for me was the *Emmanuelle* series, launched in 1974, where Dutch actress Sylvia Kristel wandered the world having guiltless bisexual adventures. So how in Aphrodite's name did second-wave feminism, born when Betty Friedan co-founded the National Organization for Women in 1967, manage to position itself against the sexual revolution? Well, it's simple: instead of encouraging women to take ownership of their own sexuality, their dogma locked onto a dead-end rhetoric of male oppression and female victimhood.
>
> After some initial resistance from a few prominent male writers, men essentially fled underground on feminist issues and now, in the absence of intelligent critique, it's been unable to self-correct ever since [which is where we are today].

Wow, that's an instant cure for priapism right there. Mercifully, she refrains from saying 'I told you so.'

Two decades earlier, Paglia predicted the current climate when she said, 'leaving sex to the feminists is like letting your dog vacation at the taxidermist'. A little harsh? Maybe. Last time I checked, plenty of feminists enjoyed sex. Then again, there are certainly some 'interesting' quotes about this from the sisterhood. America lawyer Catherine MacKinnon once said, 'All heterosexual intercourse is rape because women, as a group, are not strong enough to give meaningful consent', whilst Valerie Solanas – the woman who tried to kill Andy Warhol and penned the SCUM manifesto, which cheerfully encouraged the extermination of boys – said, 'To call a man an animal is to flatter him; he's a machine, a walking dildo.'

Thankfully, Solanas's plan died with her in 1988 and the Society for Cutting Up Men never really bounced back, but when you consider sex to be the single most dynamic, vital interchange between the genders, her choice of target isn't remotely surprising. Sex *is* power.

For some contemporary 'sextremists', the very act of it – the physical process of an erect penis entering a vagina, an anus, a mouth – isn't a natural expression of attraction, but remains proof of men's aggressive nature. Even when it's nothing of the kind. Still, in these instances, biology is begrudged for its perceived anatomical slight against women and the penis suddenly doubles as a lethal weapon (well, when it's not too small or too soft, I assume).

Ms magazine's Robin Morgan once said (and never retracted) that 'rape exists any time sexual intercourse occurs when it has not been initiated by the woman', which makes me wonder why she married a man and how she's coping with having a son. After all, Andrea Dworkin – who seemingly had a chip on each shoulder to balance herself out – once claimed: 'The annihilation of a woman's personality, individuality, will and character is the prerequisite to male sexuality … [and] every woman's son is her potential betrayer. The inevitable rapist or exploiter of another woman.'

Yep, that's *you* she's talking about there. And to think this shit still gets taught in Women's Studies classes.

But, hang on, if men weren't men – if they didn't find women attractive and want to sleep with them – what would become of all that famous feminine mystique? The power women possess as sexual beings? That timeless, intoxicating allure men are programmed to respond to? Well, quite frankly, it'd become redundant – creating millions of female eunuchs overnight. Suddenly, all over the world, girlfriends would become the butt of impotency jokes because their power to control men with sex would end.

As the gatekeepers to sex – the bouncers on the bedroom door, perhaps – they understand that, contrary to popular perception, they're not passive, weak and one-dimensional in the exchange. They're actually the ones in control because they determine when men get it. Therefore, if they play it shrewdly – both personally and politically – they can ultimately control men to their advantage.

Think about it: sex isn't something men do to women, it's an act that's enjoyed together. But politically, there's no sway in that – and, if power comes from being vulnerable, they need an oppressor. That's why men are constantly depicted as walking fragments of the patriarchy, not free-thinking individuals: it elevates women's ranking in the hierachy of marginalised groups. This, in turn, gives them status and moral superiority via the state. It maintains the myth that men are bad, women are good, which tilts the PR axis in their favour.

Meanwhile, the same women will happily use their 'erotic capital' – heels, make-up, push-up bras – to get what they want from men on a personal level. Why else do you think they dress in certain ways? To look and feel good, yes, but also to hypnotise. To have men fall at their feet. You see, a beauty that blinds is a power like no other. Something men can't replicate or get from other men, which is why there's so much fierce competition around women who want to be the source of it. Visit any northern city on a Saturday night and see for yourself. There'll be scores of them walking around with no coats on, even if it's freezing, because no time must be wasted with clothes that conceal. That would hide their magic and give rivals an advantage.

Combined, this two-pronged attack targets male sexuality from both sides – on the one hand instilling guilt and shame, on the other offering release and vanity. What's left in the middle is the increasingly narrow space where it can exist, and be expressed, freely. Then again, to keep it all going, even this orbits around a core, unspoken belief that failing to find women attractive is *the ultimate male shame*.

People pretend this isn't true, but it is. Why else do you think closeted men in Hollywood sign up for lavender marriages? Because a man who comes out socially neuters women. Rationally, of course, these women understand it doesn't matter – but subconsciously, primitively in terms of human instinct and fantasy, which Hollywood trades on, there's an unspoken disconnect. A rejection. These men have nothing to offer at the box office because they have nothing to offer in the bedroom.

Yes, OK, the film industry is mostly managed by men on an administrative level, but not really. It's actually run by money. The money women spend. I personally know an A-list actor who's gay – one who's currently plastered over London's buses because he's the lead star in a major motion picture – but experts in LA still forbid him from coming out, even though everybody in the industry knows, because it'd be professional suicide. The roles would slip away. Not as a result of horrible homophobic men, which is just one huge heterosexist prejudice, but because women have no power in that exchange. And, for them, that's a turn-off.

This is why women don't enjoy gay male porn: because it means watching their obsoleteness right there on screen. It's the same reason why straight men are conditioned to dislike gay guys. Everybody assumes it's because they fear getting hit on – but that awkwardness, which is taught, can be between a father and a son. The fear isn't sex. It's the societal downgrading men get when they don't fancy women.

'Ah, but women love the gays!' you'll say. In some ways, yes, they do – because they cannot compete for a straight man's attention. But ask her to date an openly bisexual man in the real world and I'd happily bet £100 the answer is no.

Therefore, men can wield so much more personal power if they get wise to it all and play the player. The reason gay men have more freedom to sexually express themselves than straight men is because they're not adhering to women's rules. The more heterosexual men understand this, the more control they can possess over their own sexuality – both politically and personally.

After all, they're born with the same bodies, brains and biological drive for sex, yet approach it so differently. Gay men need not justify drinking in bars with go-go dancers, parkland cruising or sex saunas, whilst Grindr was downloaded a million times long before straight, single colleagues were obsessing over Tinder. Sex can be central to a gay man's life and, religious cranks aside, he isn't vilified for it. It's never considered oppressive or sinister, just hedonistic. Straight men, however, have a very different experience. Yet the only variable between them, to put it crudely, is their partner's anatomy – meaning male sexuality only becomes 'bad' when it involves a woman.

'It's all about politics,' says Joe Kurt, expert therapist and sexologist.

> I'm constantly coaching straight guys to be more direct with their partners, like gay men. So many of them feel shame – either because their wives shame them or they've got their own self-loathing from society – but, either way, they've stopped advocating for their own sexuality. They stop talking. Instead, they secretly watch porn or cheat. These men need to feel more confident about the things they have a sexual interest in, whilst women need to learn that a man's sexual expression is equally valid.
>
> Rather than being judged for it, men should expect

curiosity and empathy in the same way their girlfriends
do. This should be a dialogue, not a monologue.

When I relay this to American female porn director Nica
Noelle, she agrees. 'The sense of shame, both private and
public, attached to sex is a very complex, multi-layered
syndrome that affects both men and women, but male
sexuality is certainly viewed as far more negative and dangerous,' she says. 'What amazes me is that no one really
challenges this view, including men. They've become so
browbeaten they're willing to accept almost anything
women say about them.'

For guys at university, this approach is increasingly
institutionalised. On the campuses of American colleges,
for example, young men are automatically assumed to
be a threat if they're sexually active.

'Reported rapes and sexual assaults reached a high
point [on campuses] in the mid-1990s,' the *Washington
Examiner*'s Ashe Schow tells me.

> At the time, women faced an uphill battle to bring their
> attackers to justice. They were told that if there was no
> blood, bruises or broken bones then they couldn't have
> been raped. This led to a national movement to correct
> that injustice, but has since evolved into an overcorrection
> – where accusers are believed outright and the accused

has to figure out a way to prove them wrong. And, even if they're exonerated, chances are their lives are still ruined.

One recent case is Peter Wu, who was expelled from New York's Vassar College after losing his virginity to a fellow student, whose father is on the staff roll. Court documents describe the incident as 'clearly consensual activity' (she sent him a Facebook message the next day saying she 'had a wondeful time'). Yet, despite being a non-native English speaker, he wasn't allowed a legal representative to present his defence at the college hearing, which subsequently destroyed his academic career. He's now suing them for damages.

Max Fraad-Wolf suffered a similar fate there. He was not allowed to be accompanied by parents or a lawyer when he was randomly summoned before a parallel criminal justice system made up of school officials, who later expelled him for sleeping with a girl – even though he was never formally charged with an offence.

Sadly, there are countless other examples. Too many to list here.

'Worryingly, I don't see this trend ending any time soon,' Ashe adds.

If modern feminism can succeed in making colleges and universities a de facto court system, why wouldn't they take that victory to the population at large? I believe we will soon see a movement to change the definition of rape and sexual assault in the criminal justice system. And, if the college definitions of 'consent' are applied to the general public, then any man in the country could find himself accused. I've considered this outcome and realised that if such a broad definition is applied to the general public, then I could accuse any man I've ever dated of sexual assault. Of course I would never do that, but it's a frightening possibility.

For a new generation of young boys, shades of this threat start early.

From childhood, they are painted as eternal predators whom girls should fear. Only last year a boy was suspended from school in America for kissing a girl on her hand – a gesture later deemed sexual harassment, irrespective of the fact he was six years old and too young to have sex. In a similar case, another boy was said to have committed 'sexual misconduct' after his peers goaded him into playfully, and momentarily, pulling his trousers down. The so-called 'charge' remains on his record.

Like a thousand pin pricks of disapproval, these messages, even if absorbed through osmosis, form a braille in the brain which reads: male sexuality is inherently bad. Over time, boys and young men internalise this, where it manifests in various hushed ways that seem unique to us, but are actually felt by most men.

A friend of mine recently confessed after much-needed reassurance, that, as a boy, he worried about being a paedophile because, like him, the girl he fancied in 1988 was also eight years old. Another is so paranoid about what constitutes 'enthusiastic consent' that he asks women to record proof as a voice memo on his phone. Then there's the mate who, on becoming a new dad, said he was uncomfortable changing his daughter's nappy because he's so over-conditioned to second-guess masculinity. It was only when his wife absolved him of this that he could relax.

Gentlemen, ENOUGH.

For centuries we've been wading through the shame associated with sex to try to reach a place of peace and resolve, rather than endless, exhausting, tail-chasing guilt. Please, for fuck's sake – and I mean that literally – let's not go back there. It offers no solution. Especially as there are already a hundred different man-shaped concerns regarding sex: Will I be good enough? Am I big enough? Will I get it up? Will I keep it up? Will I make her come – or will she fake it? And will she publicly evaluate my performance anyway? It's a minefield.

Hence if this book came with a sound-effect button, it would elicit applause right now, because – in spite of all the above – we actually do a pretty good job. Not least because the insidious assumptions about male sexuality are toxic. Which is why it's important to remember that women are not on a sexual pedestal – ever.

But let's not stop there. With the help of some world-renowned experts, here are a few more dignity-restoring facts which debunk the common myths about our sex lives:

1) MEN REACH THEIR SEXUAL PEAK AT EIGHTEEN

Some myths, like cockroaches after a nuclear war, seem to live on no matter how much we try to kill them. One of these is the frequently repeated, rarely substantiated claim that men enjoy their sexual peak at eighteen, whilst women get theirs at around fifty.

This might seem innocent enough, but don't be fooled. What it's really saying is that guys go downhill the moment they officially become men, which is con-venient, whereas women get to spend their lives forever ascending the sex scale on the carnal equivalent of a Stannah stairlift – steadily moving up without actually doing anything. Just getting up in morning means they've graduated from Kylie pre-Michael Hutchence to Kylie post-Michael Hutchence, like a modern-day Sandy from *Grease*. Thus, if we want to stay in the game and not be cuckolded by a virile teen with Herculean powers, we'd better shape up. 'Cause they need a man etc.

No need to ask why perfectly healthy men who get erections at the drop of a hat are still buying Viagra online to maintain a mythical level of performance.

So what's the truth? 'The idea that men peak sexually at eighteen originates from the belief that hormone levels reach their apex in the teen years, but that's not true,' says Vanessa Marin, a California-based sexual psychotherapist.

> Hormone levels don't dip until much later in life, and excessive hormones don't necessarily translate to amazing sex anyway.
>
> Technique and confidence improve greatly as you age, and most people report that sex feels more enjoyable as they get older. When most men look back at the sex they were having when they were eighteen, they laugh.

2) ONLY WOMEN FAKE IT

Great news, guys. We fake it too.

OK, it might not be *great* news, because somebody, somewhere, is having bad sex, but it's excellent in the sense that it's a leveller. After years of endless put-downs about our performance, it turns out women don't always get it right either.

A recent online poll at AskMen.com surveyed 50,000 people on their bedroom antics and generated some surprising results: a third of men faked it every time. Similar research conducted by *Time Out* found a matching trend in New York, whilst a local University of Kansas study reached the same conclusion. Harvard University professor Dr Abraham Morgentaler even published a book about it, called *Why Men Fake It: The Totally Unexpected Truth about Men and Sex*.

Unsurprisingly, the nagging question most people ask is: how on earth can men convincingly fake it – isn't there proof? Not necessarily. If you're wearing a condom you can quickly dispose of the evidence (or lack of), whilst without one a woman can hardly evaluate the amount of semen in her body.

Some bruised egos aside, this nifty little revelation might be a good thing, especially if it re-distributes a sexual responsibility men have single-handedly shouldered for years. Now nobody can afford to lay back and assume that dissatisfaction isn't mutual – it is.

The sexual revolution certainly kick-started a change in how men and women fuck. Now, thanks to this latest revelation, it might just come full-circle. Or, at the very least, just come.

3) WOMEN CAN HAVE MULTIPLE ORGASMS, BUT MEN CAN'T

Wrong.

Like those Magic Eye pictures, the hidden suggestion here isn't obvious, but it's this: women's bodies are complex and intricate, whilst ours are push-and-go.

The truth? Men and women can both enjoy multiple orgasms. Back in the '70s, research couple William Hartman and Marilyn Fithian studied hundreds of willing participants for their book *Any Man Can* and found that, once they got the hang of it, men could do it just as much as women. The key, if you're interested, is separating orgasm from ejaculation, which is controlled by separate nerve pathways. Sound too good to be true? Don't be so sure.

'Oh, it's true,' says Dr Beverly Whipple, a long-standing researcher recommended by the Kinsey Institute.

> In my very own lab we documented a man who was capable of multi-orgasms and multi-ejaculations during the same erection over thirty-six minutes. Now, I teach a class that shows others how to do it too. I tell them how to contract their pelvic floor muscles at the point of ejaculatory inevitability so they can keep going as long as they want. I even show them how to evaluate their muscle strength by lifting a tissue with their erection, then

– progressively, over time – a face cloth, hand towel, then
bath towel. After this, weights can be added for extra
resistance. It can really change a man's experience.

That said, this doesn't mean you now need to invest hours
trying to master it – simply having the option might be
enough. As is knowing that we aren't operating at some
kind of sex handicap to women.

4) MEN SHOULD HAVE SEX LIKE WOMEN, NOT MEN

We hear this all the time: men are crude, mechanical and
goal-driven, whereas women operate more lovingly – which
we should try to emulate. But, hang on a minute, as Lady
Gaga once astutely observed – aren't we born this way?

It seems so. Whilst men and women have the same levels of oxytocin (the chemical produced during sex which
brings people together and bonds them in intimacy),
men have higher levels of testosterone and vasopressin,
which are released after orgasm. When this happens it
causes them to distance themselves from their partner,
so whilst women want to cuddle and enjoy the afterglow,
it's because their oxytocin rush hasn't been interrupted.
Meanwhile, ours has. This isn't good or bad, just different.

And different by intelligent design, too.

'This idea of innate "goodness" in women and innate "baseness" in men is one of the most emotionally destructive feminist fairy tales,' says Dr Tara J. Palmatier, a psychologist who specialises in male therapy.

'Many of the men I work with complain their relationships lack emotional intimacy because their wives or girlfriends treat them like human dildos,' she adds. 'Men should just have sex however they want to as long as it's with another consenting adult – just like women.'

After all, sex was an act of equality long before the Equality Act.

5) PORN IS A MANIFESTATION OF SEXISM AND CAPITALISM, WHICH WOMEN NEVER WATCH OR ENJOY

There's a lot of snobbery around porn, but the taboo truth is that women enjoy two strangers fornicating in a badly lit studio just as much as we do. For exactly the same reason: it gets them off.

'At sixteen I believed everything politicians like Claire Short were saying about porn – that it was degrading to women and was dangerous, but I soon realised their anger was envy. I soon knew exploring my own sexuality was the answer, not thwarting men's freedoms,' says Dr Anna Arrowsmith, the UK's first female porn director. She cut her teeth at Central Saint Martins College of Art and Design – yes, the one Jarvis Cocker references in Pulp's 'Common People' – before moving to LA, where she now lives with her husband.

'Pornography is not the acting out of politics. It's the acting out of imagination,' she explains, trashing the suggestion that explicit material makes men sexually violent.

> Porn is a bit like professional boxing. A theorist might try and link it with street violence by arguing men see it on TV, then go out and assault someone, but we know boxing adheres to certain legal and cultural rules which render it different to everyday violence. It's a sport. People can enjoy boxing as entertainment but still appreciate that it's wrong to physically attack somebody. It's the same with porn.

Good point. But isn't it harmful to young women? Doesn't it make them need to act like porn stars with their boyfriends when actually they might just crave closeness? 'No! Research shows girls in Australia, America and the UK aren't being sexually corrupted by porn as is often suggested – in fact, they're increasingly waiting longer to lose their virginity, having their first sexual experience with a steady partner and regularly using condoms.'

So, hang on, are we saying porn actually has virtues?

Yes. First of all, it keeps couples together. Men tend to have a higher sex drive than women, so porn allows them to sate this without affairs, pestering or paying for sex. Porn also democratises the body because there's a market for anything. Half the industry is amateur, which shows all physical types. I often say to women who don't like something about themselves – body hair, for example – to stick it in a search engine and add the word porn. They'll find a host of sites which think it's the most attractive thing about them.

It also pays the wages of countless tax-payers and helps people learn about the body in the absence of good sex education. Oh, and it's the only industry I know were a woman's period is a good reason to reschedule a shoot date.

Porn is great for both women and men but, more than anything, it's a freedom of choice to be upheld.

This is particularly true with the state breathing down our necks, but the solution can simply be to see through the moral panic. The rule of thumb, or thumb and forefinger, or complete surround grip, is that it only needs to be legal and please you.

Just don't shake my hand if we ever meet.

6) IF A WOMAN DOESN'T ORGASM, IT'S YOUR FAULT

Ever since the pill dropped in the '60s, women have expected men to deliver orgasms on demand. But, in reality, loads of women struggle to climax even when they're masturbating, so gentlemen, please, relax.

Sometimes, it's them – not you.

'For a variety of reasons, women have a much harder time taking responsibility for their own pleasure than men,' says Vanessa Marin.

> Many expect their partner to make them orgasm, even if they've never been able to make themselves orgasm, which creates a whole slew of problems.
>
> As a sex therapist, I operate from the belief that we're each responsible for our own orgasms. Yes, we should all be invested in ensuring our partner is having a good time, but it's not the man's responsibility to make sure they orgasm. This can be an unpopular opinion with some women, but it's true.

Female orgasm tends to take much longer than male orgasm, and can be quite nuanced. If women explored their bodies and sexualities more, they would be able to learn what they needed to orgasm and would probably put less pressure on men to figure it all out.

7) SIZE MATTERS

My MailOnline nickname is Samantha Prick, as in 'women hate me for being pretty' Samantha Brick, because I'm often writing penis-related stories. So, to avoid repeating myself, I'm going to keep it short here – pardon the pun.

As the dedicated chapter already notes, there can be absolutely no intelligent study of penis size without a corresponding one about vaginas. If clever, board-certified researchers haven't yet twigged that the two are critically linked when it comes to sexual satisfaction then, seriously, they're in the wrong job.

Size matters – but only when there's a mismatch. Even then, this is a preference, which means both partners are equally to credit/blame* (*delete as appropriate) for the friction of their frisson.

'If a man says he prefers thin women, he's accused of

being shallow and fat-shaming. If he states a preference for large breasts, he's accused of objectifying women and worse,' adds Dr Palmatier.

> Yet, when women try to shame, humiliate and hurt men by belittling the size of his penis, it's often a socially acceptable source of amusement. This is yet another double standard when it comes to the sexes. Some women prefer a larger penis, some women prefer an average size penis. Some prefer smaller than average. Most do not care. What matters is that they're attracted to or love the man. Most women do not climax from vaginal penetration anyway. Therefore, it's more important that the couple be able to communicate what techniques, pressure, clitoral stimulation, positions etc. are most likely to result in orgasm.

This is something Dr Beverly Whipple agrees with – and has been saying for years. 'Size isn't important, but position is,' she says.

> What counts is the angle. The positions that seem to stimulate women most inter-vaginally, because they hit on the Gräfenberg spot [the G-spot, to you and me], are: woman on top, rear entry with the penis going through the vaginal wall and, thirdly, the missionary position,

but with the man kneeling up and the woman's legs over his shoulders.

8) STRIP BARS ARE HARMFUL AND DEGRADING

It's no wonder we go to strip bars: nobody talks there. Forget the semi-naked women; we go there for a bit of peace away from all the ear-bashing we get about them. Of which there's a lot.

From an objector's point of view, the argument is that they're the bastard child of misogyny and commerce. Having once been invited to one of Peter Stringfellow's venues, with – bizarrely – Rula Lenska, I could see evidence of neither. But still. If lap dancers themselves were protesting the existence of these places, then, fair enough, it would be a no-brainer – that would be slavery, which is slightly different. But these women are not bears in cages. We do not need Abraham Lincoln with his Emancipation Proclamation to roll up at the door.

Organisations like We Consent already represent people in the sex industry who exert their right to choose, politely telling others to mind their own damn business.

So perhaps the real, unspoken objection is that these women are crossing a feminist picket line. Ultimately, it's hard to say, but actress Lena Dunham recently said that part of being a feminist is giving other women the space to make choices you don't necessarily agree with. Nicely put.

'I've always been an enthusiastic supporter of strip clubs, which I view as pagan shrines for the worship of female sexual beauty and energy,' adds Camille Paglia, no doubt causing a global axis tilt from the butterfly effect of a million men nodding – very suddenly – at once.

> In 1994, I did a feature for *Penthouse* magazine where a woman reporter accompanied me to several New York venues of various socio-economic levels to demonstrate how sexist and false movie portrayals of them have been. Stripping is a legitimate genre of dance with an ancient history and should be respected as such. It's the same with the men's magazines. I support all legal softcore and hardcore pornography. It tells the primitive raw truth about sexual desire.

So there you go, it's official: male sexuality, like female sexuality, is good as standard. One is no better than the other, both are equally capable – and open to misuse.

Now that's sorted, let's get back to what nature intended – without apology. It's not making a stand for sexism or mistreating women, but for the right to enjoy sex like consenting, law-abiding, shame-free adults should.

MARRIAGE:
THE FRAUD OF THE RINGS

THERE ARE SOME GENIUS PUNS out there: the bathroom decorator who calls his company Bonnie Tiler, the bakers trading as Bread Zeppelin and the Asian restaurant named Thai Tanic, which surely goes down well – boom, boom. Then there's removal man Vanny Devito, the Tree Wise Men horticulturalists and American pancake diner I Feel Like Crepe, which are all good. Very good.

But none are better than The Fraud of the Rings for describing marriage, because – for men everywhere – that's exactly what it is. What was once the best excuse for a knees-up is now the foreplay to a sexless relationship, a painful divorce and a morbidly obese legal bill.

Yes, OK, maybe that's overstating it. There are still plenty of guys happy to take women up the aisle, as it were, but the facts speak for themselves: marriage stats across the West have nosedived in recent decades – a trend which shows no sign of slowing down. Adding to the quagmire, couples who do get hitched fail at a rate of 42 per cent, which – as Prince would say – is a sign o' the times. In fact, matrimony isn't just ailing, it's dying out faster than the average iPhone battery, which is fast.

The explanation for this is surely a complex combination of decline in religion, increase in materialism and relaxed attitudes to tradition, right? Yes and no. These are all contributing factors. As is the fact women are frequently educated above men, but rarely marry 'beneath' them – whatever that means. But there's also a more controlled, quietly anarchic reason for it all: the fact that, subconsciously or not, men are on a marriage strike. And it's growing.

A 2011 study by the PEW research centre, the American equivalent of YouGov, found that fewer young men are willing to get tied down. On the flip side, the share of young women aged eighteen to thirty-four who listed wedded bliss as a priority has risen by almost a tenth. In 1997 it was over a quarter, now it's nudging 40 per cent. Yet, for men, the opposite is true. It dropped from 35 to 29 per cent.

In online forums this is referred to, rather unimaginatively, as 'men going their own way'. It's happening everywhere from Cork to Casablanca, with single blokes saying thanks but no thanks to the old ball and chain. This doesn't happen with any great fanfare – they don't put it on a T-shirt or tattoo it onto their foreheads. They simply step back and opt out, which is precisely why it's so effective. It's stealth.

Which begs the neon-lit question: why? And should we be joining them? I put this to American academic Dr Helen Smith, who wrote the eyebrow-raising *Men on Strike: Why Men Are Boycotting Marriage, Fatherhood and the American Dream – and Why It Matters.*

'There are people out there who say men don't marry because they're immature or commitment-phobic,' she explains over the phone from Knoxville, Tennessee, with her sexy, southern drawl. Think Jerry Hall but with intonation. 'But they're all wrong – men aren't acting irresponsibly when they refuse to marry, they're acting *rationally.*'

Married with a daughter, Smith is qualified to comment

in every sense. She earned a master's degree from New York's City University before relocating south, becoming a specialist in male social psychology, and running a local clinic.

'Look, I can say this because I'm a woman,' she adds.

> But the rewards for men in modern-day marriage and fatherhood are a lot less than they used to be, yet the cost and dangers are a lot higher. Who would want to sign up for that? Ultimately, these men know there's a good chance they'll lose their friends, their respect, their space, their sex life, their money and, if it all goes wrong, their kids. They also appreciate now that single life is better than ever, so where's the incentive? Men aren't wimping out by staying unmarried, they're being smart. They don't want to enter into a legal contract with somebody who could effectively take half their savings, pension and property when the honeymoon period is over.

Crikey, that all sounds a bit bleak.

Let's look at the proof: in 2009 the Office for National Statistics released figures showing that marriage is at its lowest level since 1895. In England and Wales there were 286,634 ceremonies during 2011, which is almost a whopping 50 per cent freefall from 1972, when almost 480,285 couples tied the knot. Enter stage left: a slew of young women looking for Mr Right and frequently being unable to find him.

Nowhere does this manifest more than in the world of online dating. Match-making sites have never been more prolific – and profitable – than they are today, with an estimated annual industry turnover of £2 billion. There's Match, Guardian Soulmates, Plenty of Fish, Tinder, My Single Friend, E-Harmony, Lovestruck and Hello Cupid to name a few. But what do many of these sites have in common? Yep, more women actively looking for marriage in their profiles than men.

Clearly, something is amiss.

So, what gives? Well, the short answer is: us. We give. Everything. Or at least it seems that way. A quick glance at any high-profile divorce over the last few years shows it's husbands, not wives, who get hit hardest in a separation. Agreed, we're dealing in sweeping generalisations here, but it remains the rule, rather than the exception.

Check out these real-life adverts for remaining a bachelor: when British businessman Alan Miller wed his first wife Melissa in 2003, he thought it was forever. She immediately decided to give up work, including her £85,000 salary, to become what was dubbed a 'Harvey Nichols wife', which meant spending her time shopping, lunching and spending – an impressive lifestyle for someone who doesn't earn a living. When they separated just two years and nine months later, he was forced to pay her a £5 million divorce sum which included his £2.3 million home in Chelsea and a separate £2.7 million lump sum – despite the fact they had no children. That equates to more than £6,000 per day. Ker-ching!

He argued, rather brilliantly, that he would've been better off if he'd knocked her down in his car and had to pay compensation but the Court of Appeal said that by marrying her he'd given his wife 'an expectation of a significantly better standard of living' – something he must maintain to make her happy, at his expense. For-ever. Because he's a man.

Kenneth MacFarlane, one of the big boys at accounting firm Deloitte, suffered a similar fate. He had to give his ex-wife his luxury home and £250,000 every year for life because he worked full-time during their relationship. She even went back to court for a second bite of the cherry when he was later given a pay-rise. A ruling which makes Paul McCartney's judgment seem almost fair. When the Beatles star married Heather Mills in 2002, the world winced at what was effectively a six-year, slow-motion car crash. Unsurprisingly, Mills quickly got pregnant and – when the inevitable divorce came through – got her hands on £24.3 million. Experts say he was lucky. If he hadn't roped in family law guru Fiona Shackleton the figure could've been more like £200 million.

Love me do? Love me don't, more like.

For all its pulling power, it seems the concept of marriage has – ironically – been adulterated by big-money pay-outs and, to quote Kanye West for a bit of gangster credibility, a generation of gold diggers. So, sorry, Beyoncé, it's little wonder we won't put a ring on it, even if we do like it. Besides, it's not just 'a' ring, these days, but two. One for popping the question, the other for sealing the deal.

Forget any idea that this is about tradition or romance, it's actually just good old-fashioned marketing.

Before the 1930s there was no such thing as buying an engagement ring for a future spouse. People got married because they wanted to, rather than because the bloke begged with a box on bended knee. This was only kick-started in 1938, when jewellery company De Beers began running ads which said 'real' men (read: ignore this and she'll think you're a dud) bought their fiancées expensive rings to prove their worth. In a media masterstroke, this set a behavioural code which – funnily enough – also generated a tonne of profit. Not least because they ruled – in a vulgar example of commercial profit-chasing – that the average ring should cost two months' salary.

The laughable part? Years later, De Beers chairman himself, Nicky Oppenheimer, admitted that diamonds 'are intrinsically worthless' – which is surprisingly true.

The only reason they're expensive to shoppers is because De Beers have a monopoly on diamond mining and up the price by restricting supply, hence marking up the retail price. In other words: it's a great big fucking scam. Which is yet another reason to either a) stay away from marriage altogether and focus on having healthy relationships – kept healthy by the nagging reality that it could all end at any time – or b) buy your bling from Argos. For richer or poorer and all that.

Then again, even being economical isn't enough. In 2011, a US appeals court in Georgia ordered a man to pay $50,000 to his one-time fiancée for calling off their wedding. Melissa Cooper sued Christopher Ned Kelley for fraud and breach of promise after their ten-year relationship ended. In a similar case, Florida woman RoseMary Shell successfully sued her ex-fiancé, Wayne Gibbs, for $150,000 after he dumped her in 2007. She argued that his promise of marital bliss was tantamount to a binding contract. Naturally, she won, despite the fact he'd already paid off $30,000 of *her* debts whilst they were together (and he only called off the wedding when he discovered she had lots more).

Christ, only in America – right?

Well, not quite. India is enjoying its own through-the-looking-glass approach to tying the knot. Currently, divorce can be filed as 'no fault' by either partner – but only wives have the right to oppose it. They also automatically get half of the bloke's property list – whether currently owned or due for inheritance – whilst her landlord portfolio remains off the table. Meanwhile, over in Australia, there's a 'Mistress Law' whereby a married man's assets can now readily be accessed by the other woman. In a breakthrough test case, the bit-on-the-side told press: 'I gave him the best years of my life. He always told me he would look after me, then he left me. I had committed myself fully to him for all those years. So this is also about giving our relationship a validity.'

Er, forget validity. This is about punishment and female self-entitlement. Why couldn't she look after herself like every other adult on the planet?

I put this radical theory to Suzanne Venker, journalist, author and professional feather-ruffler. Speaking to me from St Louis, she tells me in no uncertain terms that the problem is women wanting to have their cake and eat it. See, I told you she was controversial.

'We messed with the old marriage structure and now it's broken,' she says

> Back in the day, stay-at-home mothers got a financial reward in divorce settlements because child-rearing doesn't pay cash, which was fair – that's an option afforded to women by working husbands. It's teamwork.

Now, we want total independence from men, but if we divorce one – even without having kids – we still expect to get alimony forever. We can't have it both ways.

This, along with bridezillas and the prospect of endless domestic criticisms, is exactly why we're saying 'I don't' rather than 'I do'. Men need marriage like a fish needs a bicycle.

'Many women have been raised to think of men as the enemy,' Venker adds:

It's precisely this dynamic – women good, men bad – that has destroyed the relationship between the sexes. After decades of browbeating, men are tired. Tired of being told there's something fundamentally wrong with them. Tired of being told that if women aren't happy, it's men's fault. The 'rise' of women has not threatened men. It has pissed them off.

Maybe she has a point. In one way, the appeal of marriage is like old VHS tapes. We look at them via our childhood with a warm, nostalgic glow. Almost through a sepia-toned Instagram filter. But deep down we know the quality was always a bit shit – you'd be ten minutes into *The Goonies* (which you had to watch that night or face a fine) and be stuck manually adjusting the tracking, which didn't make a difference anyway. Yet people had faith in it because it was the best option they had. And big money fuelled the fire. Blockbuster was one of the biggest business models in its sector – it was a tent pole in home rental movie revenue. But suddenly, without warning, the bottom fell out of the market. Change happened. Ideas developed, thinking shifted. People wanted greater convenience. First, this came in the form of DVDs – something lighter, faster and more understated – which, at the risk of battering a metaphor to death, is what marriage experienced with registry offices. They were modernised, compact, less-is-more. Then, like blu-ray or special edition boxsets, they too became pimped, like eloping to Gretna Green or drive-thru chapels in Las Vegas.

Still, behind all the clever technology and shiny, new rebranding remained an ageing transaction. People were still asked to buy.

Eventually, like the free love philosophy of the '60s, LoveFilm ditched that altogether, meaning that, with new technology, we didn't even need to leave the house to get what we wanted (although I'm saying absolutely nothing about mail-order brides here). More recently, the once leading concept behind Blockbuster was boiled down to live streaming on Netflix, which created a game-changer when it simply allowed entertainment – read: pleasure – to be enjoyed on demand.

Today, people don't just want this in relation to the small stuff, but across the board. Less restriction and more freedom. Fewer penalties, more value for money. They want a life that's high definition, good quality and convenient, without endless, disproportionate financial penalties for putting their tape in somebody else's machine.

Ironically, even in Hollywood, where all these dreams are bought and sold, marriage rarely ends well. Actor Robin Williams wed/divorced twice in good faith but – despite working solidly for decades – faced near-financial ruin after both separations cost him an estimated $30 million in settlements. In a bid to offset the damage, he ended up coming out of retirement at the age of sixty-two to work full-time on TV series *The Crazy Ones*, but we all know how that ended. 'Divorce is expensive. I used to joke they were going to call it "all the money", but they changed it to "alimony",' he mused. 'It's ripping your heart out through your wallet.'

Yet, by Tinsel Town standards, divorce is still a credible career move. Look at Goldie Hawn's film *The First Wives Club*. Billed as a family comedy about rinsing your ex for all he's worth, it's actually just a group of women prostituting themselves with the backing of the law. The moral of the immoral story? Men are untapped resources to be extracted, like crude oil in Texas. Girls: dig in and strike rich.

But when women leave their husbands in films such as *The Hours* or *Thelma and Louise*, it's all good. They're heroines. Even when the men do nothing wrong.

OK, these are just movies – I get it. But it captures an ethos. A cultural trend. A way of thinking around men, their industriousness and their money.

Look at former Arsenal footballer Ray Parlour. When he married girlfriend Karen in 1998, it all started out rosy, as it always does. But, by the time it fell apart in 2004, the former optician's nurse didn't just get two mortgage-free houses, £38,500 in annual support for their three children and a £250,000 tax-free lump sum. Oh no, she also got personal maintenance of £406,500 from his *future* earnings too. This, she argued, is because she 'encouraged' him to be a good midfielder.

He shoots, she scores, you might say.

Which is precisely why WAG culture now rages through our country like an aggressive venereal disease. Girls of sixteen aspire to be glamorous girlfriends because it's an easy life, not because they love the game – or even the men playing it. Young women who wear so much make-up they have to tip their heads back to get their eyes open are encouraged to hunt in packs until they snag a rich footballer, who'll play, play, play to pay, pay, pay. Why? Because it beats getting up at 7 a.m., doing the daily commute and actually thinking about something other than themselves. When Pot Noodle summed this up in one of their adverts, the tag line was: 'Why try harder?' Indeed.

There's even a technical term for it: hypergamy. The act of 'marrying up' by securing a rich man. It might not be PC, but it's still real. Just ask James Taranto from the *Wall Street Journal*. According to him, it's steeped in nature. 'Any evolutionary psychologist will tell you that female hypergamy – more broadly defined as the drive to mate with dominant males – is an animal instinct,' he tells me.

But what would happen if Ray Parlour – or, let's be honest here, you – got married and divorced four times? Would he, or you, have to give all his money away to four different exes who were each capable of earning their own salary? I put this theory to Camilla Baldwin, divorce lawyer extraordinaire, who's based in Mayfair. Her no-bullshit approach has seen her hired by celebrities, sportsmen and bankers on countless multi-million-pound bloodbaths. Thankfully, she didn't charge me her standard £450 per hour rate. Further proof, in case you needed it, that marriage and divorce are financial enemas.

'The judge in Ray's case basically disliked him,' she says.

> He ordered a very, very generous reward – over and
> above what the ex-wife needed – partly because he didn't

like him. This happens all the time. Going to court is a human thing and how a person comes across flavours the way a case is decided. I'm often at the Principal Registry in London, where certain judges are known for always favouring women. Alan Miller's QC didn't like him either. It's a subconscious bias, but it's real. Judges are biased.

Hmm. Constance Briscoe, anyone?

Camilla's eponymous firm, rated one of our country's best by the *Financial Times*, has only one male lawyer in a team of fifteen because 'there aren't many men in family law', yet the bulk of her customers are husbands and fathers.

These men get married in their twenties when they leave university. Maybe it lasts for twelve years, but then it ends with them paying maintenance for the rest of their lives – even if they remarry and have more children with somebody else, which is manifestly unfair. I have several clients who have been divorced from their first wives longer than they were married to them, but these men still have to support them. It's outrageous.

The Law Commission agrees. They recently released a paper which advised limiting spousal maintenance to three years, like they do in Scotland. But don't start celebrating just yet: it's still a long way from being implemented. And, in the meantime, it's a costly nightmare.

'I've spent so much time with clients who are absolutely bonkers,' she adds.

> It often happens when you have a younger woman marrying an older man for a short period of time. I recently worked with a lovely Irish guy, seventy-two, who wed a woman in her forties. He'd made his wealth long before meeting her, and they were only married for a few months, but she still got a million pounds from him. What's sad is that she married him to divorce him – and he fell for it.

I quickly take a moment to bang my head against a brick wall, then resume the conversation. So, let me ask the impossible here: are we saying women sometimes marry for money?

'Absolutely! AB-SO-LUTELY,' she bellows down the phone.

> God, if I'd divorced somebody rich I'd be having a fine time now. I wouldn't need to work. That's how you make real money – more than the average person ever dreams of. One woman I know, a barrister, has amazing earning

potential but refuses to go over £15,000 a year because it would affect her husband's maintenance. These kinds of women are insane. It's not about equality, it's about revenge. These women hate their ex-husbands and think they're justified in avenging a broken heart by any means.

When I ask her what she – as a hard-working woman – thinks of it all, she pauses before responding.

Honestly? I always just feel so sorry for the men.

I once represented a client who'd been married to his wife for fifteen years. He was a very successful trader in the City and – without being prompted – offered his wife half of his £40 million fortune when they split, but she demanded more. She dragged him off to court, got a team of lawyers together and argued £20 million wasn't enough to re-house herself. Eventually, he gave in because he couldn't stand the litigation, but she hadn't worked a day in her life. I even said to her barrister, 'Look, this is madness. We are real people doing real jobs for nothing like the sums discussed here. How can you stand there with a straight face and make such demands?' But she won anyway.

To be fair, it's not just women. It's bigger than that. It's a wider habit of stinging men (take him to the cleaners!

etc.) for simply being male, even if everyone is supposed to be equal and self-sufficient.

Only last year I reported on the story of a man who was trying to reach a settlement with his civil partner. As part of my research I spoke with the ex's lawyer, who – in all seriousness – said that his client deserved 50 per cent of his partner's fortune because 'he'd helped decorate the apartment they shared for eighteen months', despite not actually paying any of the mortgage. No kidding. At that point I was so aghast I wanted to bite through the phone wire with my teeth with frustration, but, thankfully, I was calling from my mobile.

So, what's a guy to do? 'If a man's determined to get married then he must get a pre-nup, otherwise it's simply too expensive,' Camilla insists. 'More and more people are doing it. In fact, people are even getting post-nups now, but men must be insistent – otherwise steer clear altogether. Be in a relationship by all means, even live together, but don't get married. Especially if you have any prospect of making money.'

OK, let's park the cost of bankrolling an ex for the moment. Instead, let's look at the average price of an actual wedding. Some swift research shows they don't call it the 'big day' for nothing. Here's why: the latest stats say you'll need around £18,000 for the average 'do. This includes: the venue, the wedding dress, the rings, the photographer, the flowers, the catering, the enter-tainment, your outfit, the bridesmaids' dresses and the honeymoon.

And, even then, it might still be a shit day.

A quick counting-on-fingers calculation proves that, for the same amount, you can get: an amazing holiday with first-class flights around the world, a flash car, a deposit on an apartment, a wardrobe of suits from Savile Row or a debilitating sex addiction with high-class hookers. You could even replicate Stevie Nicks's alleged penchant for hiring somebody to anally insert your cocaine stash to avoid doing what's become known as 'a Danniella West-brook'. Whatever your preference, it has to be better than a doomed marriage if you actually *enjoy* spunking your hard-earned money up the wall.

Sadly, there's even more bad news. The quantity – and quality – of sex also dwindles after marriage. A recent vox pop of 3,000 couples found that those who had had sex four times a week before their wedding did it just once a week afterwards. Meanwhile, the majority of single-tons reported being sexually satisfied almost all the time. Which makes me wonder: is marriage even a natural state for human beings? Aren't we all just animals? Surely a visit to any branch of Tiger Tiger would confirm this.

Even France's former First Lady Carla Bruni-Sarkozy admits she's 'easily bored by monogamy' whilst Cameron

Diaz has said relationships would ideally only last 'two, five or twenty years' – not forever. So why, even when we know it probably won't have the fairy-tale ending, do we go for it anyway? Are we all just hopeless romantics – or lemmings walking off a cliff?

My next port of call is renegade anthropological researcher Christopher Ryan, who co-wrote the controversial *New York Times* bestseller *Sex at Dawn*.

'If you're asking if long-term sexual monogamy is a natural state for human beings, the answer is clearly no – at least, for most human beings,' he asserts. 'We're as attracted to novelty and variety in our sexual appetites as we are in diet, art, music, travel etc. An appetite for this is intrinsic to our intelligence and social nature.'

According to him, the body itself proves this.

> In *Sex at Dawn*, we say the external scrotum is like having a beer fridge in the garage. Any man who has a fridge full of beer is expecting a party to start any time. The external testicles are a clever way to keep sperm ready to go at a moment's notice. This is just one among many anatomical indications that our ancestors were quite promiscuous.

As he talks, I realise that perhaps what marriage really needs is a makeover. Less Jo Brand, more rebrand.

Something to make it more appealing, especially for men. So I approach Saatchi & Saatchi, one of the world's biggest advertising agencies. They famously ushered Margaret Thatcher into power in 1979 with their memorable poster campaign for the Conservative Party, which showed a dole queue snaking out of an employment office and disappearing into the skyline. The tag line read: 'Labour isn't working'.

So, let's stretch our imagination and pretend the government has offered a limitless budget to make marriage man-friendly. What tactics would they use?

'There are many commitments in life but few are for life in quite the same way as marriage,' says Richard Huntington, the company's chief strategy officer.

> Marriage means signing a blank emotional cheque and, where marriage goes, men assume kids, mortgages and weekends picking out wallpaper patterns follow. In their heads, men believe marriage is emasculating.
>
> This fear of commitment would need tackling head on, so the commitment brand would need to be relaunched. There are a number of ways we could do this. We might invoke the fear of losing her with 'if you have one foot out of your relationship, so does she'. We might challenge perceptions of the dreariness of married life by communicating that 'she is not your

wife, she is your partner in crime'. Or we might focus on the masculinity implied by having people utterly depend on you by saying that 'marriage makes a real man of you'.

Sounds like the treatment for the De Beers ad, right? That's because it is. Commercials are formulaic because they follow a formula. Advertising agencies are paid millions to manipulate the human emotions that drive us – especially fear. The fear of missing the boat. The fear of missing out. The fear of growing old and dying alone.

But – brilliantly – courage, the opposite of fear, which men have in spades, allows us to accept the reality that, no matter how much we love somebody, no matter how good our intentions are, the success of a marriage isn't just down to us. It takes two. And the overwhelming majority of divorces are filed by women. The Office of National Statistics put the rates at 66 per cent for 2011, whilst it was 72 per cent in the early 1990s.

OK, given the aforementioned jackpot settlements, this is hardly surprising. But a study sponsored by Yorkshire Building Society, which questioned 3,515 divorced adults, found that men suffer the most when it goes sour. Apparently, it makes us feel 'devastated, confused, betrayed and even suicidal; whilst women are more likely to feel relieved, liberated and happy'.

Divorced men are also more prone than women to finding solace in drinking; going back to an old toxic flame (you stopped seeing her for a reason!); and self-medicating with risky, casual sex. Adding insult to injury, they also say we worry more about finding a new partner and throw ourselves into work as a distraction.

'We're bred as children to be needy and to think we need another person to complete us. It's driven into us from an early age,' says Guy Blews, a relationship expert in Los Angeles.

> This all leads to expectation, which, as we know, is the mother of disaster. Humans aren't very good at learning to live in the moment and keep a relationship going as it started, so we try and make it permanent. We think it takes the pressure off because it's sanctioned by law, so effectively nobody else can steal them, but married people separate all the time. It's a false hope.
>
> We're also sold the lie that we're emotionally and financially more stable in a marriage, but if we boil it down to its basic truth, we only do it out of secret desperation and obligation. We fear that if we're not married by a certain age there's something wrong with us. We fear losing our girlfriends or not finding anyone else. For men, there's a big sense of obligation to propose – if only to please their partner.

He has a point. Rarely is a wedding driven by a man who wants a big day and a slow-dance to Westlife.

So, what's the answer? 'Being honest with yourself,' says Blews.

> We need to accept human nature for what it is. Infidelity is one of the main reasons people break up. That's because humans aren't really, truly designed for monogamy. Back in the caveman days everybody slept with everybody and the strongest sperm fertilised the healthiest egg. This created the best offspring. It's nature. Don't get me wrong, the idea of marriage is great, but it doesn't leave room for the gritty reality that everything changes – whether we like it or not.
>
> Funnily enough, there is no love, trust or belief in marriage because, if there was, there'd be no need for it in the first place.

'Let me put it another way,' he enthuses.

> Imagine I take you up in an aeroplane and give you a parachute. I tell you to jump, but there's a 50 per cent chance you'll die outright. There's another 40 per cent chance you'll get to the ground safely, but have a lot of broken bones. Maybe some permanent damage. Then there's an 8 per cent chance you'll get away with a few scrapes. Unfortunately,

> there's only a 2 per cent possibility of landing on your
> feet – happy and alive to tell the tale. Still want to jump?

Needless to say, as far as proposals go, that's not an attractive one.

See, calculated risks are one thing – that's what life, love and the best relationships are all about – but marriage isn't integral to any of them. It's just an expensive, unnecessary bolt-on.

Besides. at a time when we're more fashion-conscious than ever, rings on fingers aren't just a thing of the past, but also a thing of the passé. A bit like those old-fashioned VHS tapes.

And, seriously, who'd give up what they have now for one of those?

THE MALE PILL:
THE GREATEST THING
WE'VE NEVER HAD

WHEN I ENTER PROFESSOR LEE Smith's office at the University of Edinburgh's Centre for Reproductive Health, two things strike me: the stack of scientific papers on his desk and the mouse-shaped clock hanging from his wall.

'It's bespoke,' he says, pointing to the latter. 'You won't see many of these about.' Quite. The pendulum below it, swinging furiously from left to right, is designed to look like a pair of testicles. Not something you'd expect from the local Chair of Genetic Endocrinology, but, somehow, it fits.

'There's plenty of scope for fun in here,' he says, drinking coffee from a mug bearing the legend 'World's Best* Advisor' (note the disclaimer asterisk). There's also a Viagra stationery holder with very erect pens.

Science, it seems, has developed a sense of humour. And Smith, for all his myriad qualifications and breakthrough discoveries, is less boffin, more everyman – which is reassuring given that he holds our sperm in his hands – albeit metaphorically, thank God.

At just thirty-nine, Smith, with the help of his team – scientists from Scotland, England, France, China and Taiwan – has found new scope for a male pill by safely blocking a vital gene called Katnal 1, which controls an early stage in semen development. 'We work on the wider issue of male fertility and testosterone's role in the body,' he says, framed by pictures of his two children. 'But when we inadvertently found a faulty gene that made men infertile, we suddenly had the basis for a contraceptive.'

Strange how it's always little things that make big things happen.

Smith started his career in Oxford University during the late 1990s, where he worked on testes development and early sex determination – essentially, whether parents end up with a boy or a girl. Several years later, he was head-hunted for his current role in Scotland, where he now controls a £4.1 million grant from the Medical Research Council. Twenty-four months into his five-year tenure and he's already pioneering knowledge where others failed.

'One of the key issues surrounding previous male con-traception was the need to reduce testosterone in order to block sperm development altogether,' he explains. 'This can lead to unwelcome side effects such as acne and mood swings. Therefore, our non-hormonal approach, which prevents sperm development without changing testosterone levels, is a significant step forward. We now have an incredible advantage over drug development programmes.'

Reassuringly, Dr Smith's pill would allow sperm to be produced as normal, but would just inhibit them from maturing properly. Because this biological tweak is to a specific gene and not men's overall hormone balance, it would also be side effect-free (which is a marketing mas-terstroke as much as a medical one).

For a closer look, we enter the lab. 'There are some funky machines in here!' he says, proudly. Inside, it's packed with white coats, test tubes and very expensive equipment – including something called a genotyper, which spins very fast to 'run a chemical cycle that monitors gene changes'. It's everything you've seen in films, but real.

'Here's the viral suite. Don't go in there!' he warns. 'That's where we take the DNA out of viruses, swap it for something we want, then use it to infect cells. We did this recently with our mice; it switched off certain genes in their testes, so we know how to make them infertile.'

As we navigate it all, the obvious question is: why mice? 'They're a model. An inexact model, but a model all the same,' he says. 'Men aren't going to donate a testicle, but mice have the same cell types as men, the same hormones targeting certain cells and they also produce sperm. There are some structural differences, but – for the vast majority – it's a good model.' OK, fine. But how successfully could the findings repeat in us? 'In our studies with mice, we reduced sperm numbers by 89 per cent six weeks after beginning treatment – and of the remaining sperm, only 5 per cent were mobile,' he says, confidently. 'This timeframe can be doubled for men as their sperm development is slightly slower. Twelve weeks from starting treatment would be a good ball-park figure – pardon the pun. From this point, the patient wouldn't be able to father children until he stopped taking the contraceptive. Then, full fertility would resume within two months.'

Boldly, Smith then predicts the drug could be on the

market within a decade – initially as an injection, then modified into gels and oral tablets for maximum global consumption. However, this isn't a one-man race.

'There are 200 papers a day being printed on what we're doing, so it's very much the first to publish…' he adds. 'It's like a journalist breaking a story. We're all running towards the same finish line.'

Four thousand miles away in India, scientist Sujoy Guha has spent the past thirty years developing Vasalgel; a one-off injection to a man's vasa deferentia, the ducts which carry semen from the testes. This coats the inside of each tube, killing sperm as it passes through them. One shot is effective for up to a decade and can be reversed with a second jab at any time. It's now in the final stages of Indian medical and governmental approval and is on the cusp of FDA endorsement in the United States too.

Meanwhile, in a lab at Australia's Monash University, scientists are working on the mutation of a gene called RABL2. This causes sperm to grow tails that are roughly 17 per cent shorter than average, meaning they're unable to propel themselves towards a woman. 'There's truly a desperate need for more contraceptives,' says Moira O'Bryan, who's leading the study. 'Personally, I want to see a situation where every child is wanted. For many people, current contraceptive options aren't enough or don't fit their lifestyles. It's a problem.'

For men, this is particularly true. Whilst women enjoy the lion's share of choices, we have just three: condoms, vasectomy and abstinence. No prizes for guessing which comes out on top. Even then, condoms are rarely the practical ideal. They vary in comfort and fit, they can be difficult or embarrassing to get on – risking erection loss – and, crucially, they can puncture – either literally, or the romantic mood. In comparison, the female pill has been a monumental success since its launch in 1960, now being used by more than 100 million women worldwide (making a small fortune for drug companies along the way – you do the maths).

So why is our version taking so long?

Whilst the latest developments may be new, the general concept is not. In the 1970s, Brazilian endocrinologist Dr Elsimar Coutinho developed one of the first ever male pill prototypes. Made from all-natural cottonseed, it didn't go down too well with pharmaceutical companies for obvious reasons (hardly a money-spinner if the local health shop can produce a no-frills version for half the price), but it also suffered social resistance. When launched at the 1974 World Health Conference in Budapest, religious groups voiced concern and feminists staged a boycott, storming Coutinho's presentation and demanding that only women – not men – should be making choices about parenthood. How retro. Despite some compelling evidence, his vision – a bit like the Sinclair C5 – just didn't take off.

Things picked up in the mid-1990s when two pharmaceutical giants, Organon and Schering-Plough, ran their own self-financed studies, but these got sidelined when they were bought out by competitors with different agendas. It all suffered a major retrenchment until recently. So, why the resurgence?

'Every now and again we reach a dam of knowledge,' Smith says of the industry. 'Then, as more information comes in, it clicks and, together, we take a step forward. That's how science works.'

Fortunately, one previous sticking point – religious objection – has since relaxed. 'There's no reason why men would be any different to the 98 per cent of Catholic women in America who ignore the bishops' ban on birth control,' says Jon O'Brien, President of Washington-based faith group Catholics for Choice. 'The people who head the Catholic Church are obsessed with the pelvic zone,' he adds, in his ocean-hopping Irish-American accent.

'That's why our organisation exists. So when they're lobbying a UN official over family planning, we remind people to listen to the sixty million Catholic Americans who live in the real world, not the 350 US bishops who make the rules but are largely ignored.'

Now, the bigger consideration is what a pill could offer the brotherhood. For most, the answer is obvious: limitless, no-strings sex. For the first time since Eve tempted Adam with that damn apple, men would truly be empowered to control the outcome of their sexual encounters, only becoming fathers when they wanted to.

Yes, accidents happen, but the unspeakable reality of men being 'trapped' would also end overnight. Those such as Liam Gallagher, Jude Law, Hugh Grant, Steve Bing and Sacha Gervasi – the screenwriter who was stunned, then snubbed, when he got Geri Halliwell pregnant after a six-week fling – would no longer find themselves becoming fathers when all they wanted (and agreed to) was a quick shag. No more shotgun weddings, no more duped daddies, no more surprise calls from the Child Support Agency.

That said, a male contraceptive would also be good for women. The original pill is highly effective, but packed with side effects that include weight gain, DVT threat and, rather ironically, reduced libido. To offer women respite from this is, at the very least, good manners.

Contemporary US feminist Ariel Levy gave her slant. 'I would welcome it, absolutely,' she says from her Manhattan home with an east coast purr. 'I disagree with critics who claim it infringes on women's rights: I'd say it expands their options. Men and women should share the burden of contraception. The tricky thing is that we're still the ones who get pregnant, so for a woman to rely on the male pill as her only form of birth control, she needs to be in a relationship with a man she trusts pretty completely.'

True. But hang on, don't men have to trust women who say *they're* on the pill? Yes, women may carry the child physically, but it's men who carry it financially. Besides, if everyone took responsibility for themselves, wouldn't it simply mean that all pregnancies were planned by both parties – all the time?

When journalist Liz Jones famously revealed she stole her boyfriend's sperm from a used condom, despite his assertions that he had no interest in becoming a father, the nation was shocked and appalled – but only because it was finally out in the open. Let's not pretend this shit hasn't been going on for years. Fortunately, there was no baby, but her behaviour is neither new nor rare. It's a tactic of many who want a child at any cost – well, except the cost of actually going it alone.

Britain's Got Talent judge Amanda Holden recently confessed to deceiving her husband into fatherhood. Speaking to *OK!* magazine, she said, 'I've always been practical – a fixer … I had to have another baby. I know I may get criticism, but it was about survival … Men don't understand. Tricking Chris was devious – but I had to have another baby.'

Now imagine a twist of science where a man says that exact same thing about a woman's eggs. Let's assume, say, Johnny Depp sleeps with Vanessa Paradis one last time and nicks some of her eggs – then fertilises them with his semen in a lab. She then gets a legal letter outlining all the child support she'll need to provide for the next eighteen years, whilst the world puts pressure on her to 'be a real woman' and play an active role by embracing servitude – regardless of the fact her choice has been, for want of a better term, violated.

Would everybody be so laissez-faire? Would the media celebrate? Would they side with Depp as the sympathetic character – and against Paradis for not voluntarily granting him the child he so passionately craved? No way. So, if that's the case, why is it any different when it happens to men? Is it perhaps the outmoded, entitled assumption that men should simply provide, exponentially, forever – no matter what the circumstances?

Even Holden's boss, Simon Cowell, was involuntarily thrust into fatherhood thanks to Lauren Silverman. Sure, he may be happy now, but his entire life was changed by somebody else's decision. The ability to afford men control over this with a centimetre-wide tablet is nothing less than revolutionary. After all, a woman's desire to have a child is no more valid than a man's not to.

Paul Elam is a men's rights activist from Texas and the

founder of A Voice for Men. He argues that men have as much riding on pregnancy as women do in the long term, but not nearly as much control. 'The arrival of a male pill would mark the first time in history that men will be empowered to see themselves as near full participants in reproductive choices,' he says.

And it will force wider culture to see them in the same light too.

This is important because men have historically been forced into a passive role in the reproductive picture. Currently, men compete for sexual selection and wait to be chosen. When they are, they wait to be informed of any consequences. They wait to be told if the baby will be carried to term, or will be aborted. They wait to be told if they will be allowed to participate in the life of the child. They wait to be told what they will have to pay, and how much for how long, regardless of whether they want or intended to be a parent. The implied agreement when having sex is that men have no say in the outcome, and that if they don't like it they should abstain. In most areas that implied social agreement is backed by law. The male pill changes this forever because it gives men an attractive option to control the outcome of their sexual encounters.

It allows men to share the responsibility for birth

control with women, without forcing them to forsake the pleasure of sex. If the male pill fulfils its promise of effective birth control with no side effects, it also may allow women to stop taking potentially dangerous medications that pose significant risks. With both men and women having options, it means pregnancy would be a conscious choice made openly between both partners. What could be better than that?

When I put this to Rebecca Fleming, head of press at London's Family Planning Association, I hold the phone from my ear and expect fireworks. 'We actually agree with him,' she says, simpatico. 'When we talk to men, they are ideologically very supportive of contraceptive methods and managing their paternity.'

A-ha! But this isn't just about babies, is it? It's also about sexual irresponsibility and STDs. That's the snag: inadvertently creating a new generation of reckless men who'd fuck without giving a fuck.

'Actually, that's a red herring,' she says, authoritatively. 'Many women on the pill have unprotected sex *because* they're on the pill – and that hasn't stopped it being a success. It's a separate, ongoing issue and shouldn't be used to derail men's options.'

Good point. Just because the female pill controls pregnancy – and not STDs – doesn't make it any less of a huge success. Nor is it any less of a money-spinner. The same applies to a male pill.

'In fact,' Fleming says, 'countless men call the FPA's helpline because they frequently find unplanned pregnancies "devastating". Our statistics show that half of all pregnancies are unplanned. We know these can be as distressing for men as they are for women, but it only strikes men at this point. And, once a woman is pregnant, they have no say on whether she keeps it or not. The only opportunity men have to exercise choice is at the contraception stage. That's why we want to see more of them putting their reproductive needs first.'

When I ask (through gritted teeth) whether men are trustworthy enough to take a contraceptive, Fleming doesn't mess around. 'That's just absurd,' she says. 'Men do responsible things every day.'

For the sake of credibility, I request some proof. She points me in the direction of a 2008 study by GfK National Opinion Polls, which shows that 36 per cent of men would happily take a male contraceptive if available, whilst a further 26 per cent might, providing it were safe and reversible (something which would be a medical prerequisite anyway). Add these together and you have 62 per cent already on board.

Oxford Journals also published a 1999 study of 1,894 women at family planning clinics across Scotland, South

Africa and China. More than 90 per cent of those in Scotland and South Africa thought a male pill was a good idea, whilst Chinese women (71 per cent in Hong Kong and 87 per cent in Shanghai) were only slightly less positive. Reassuringly, only thirty-six people said they wouldn't trust their partner at all – that's just 2 per cent of the total.

I then approach the British Pregnancy Advisory Service – an organisation which guides women through their options around abortion. Clare Murphy, BPAS's Director of External Affairs, says men should ignore the cynics (some might call them misandrists) who say they'd be unreliable with a pill. Especially as our only other real option – the vasectomy – is increasingly unavailable on the NHS. 'After condoms, vasectomy is the sole protection for men,' she says. 'Even then, we're seeing a decline in their popularity due to funding cut-backs, so it's either not available or severely restricted. Additionally, men are also more conscious that relationships break down. If they do, they naturally want the option to start a second family elsewhere.'

In 2001/02, there were 37,700 UK vasectomies, compared with 15,106 in 2011/12. The figures have fallen 16 per cent from 2010 to 2011 alone. In the USA the scenario is even more depressing, with a man needing to get his wife's permission before doctors perform a vasectomy – otherwise they refuse.

But would the NHS even bother to prescribe a male pill if it were available? Under equality legislation, they'd probably have to, says Murphy. In fact, they'd open themselves up to litigation on the basis of gender bias if they didn't. The tricky bit, she adds, isn't legal wrangling or the fear of high-profile discrimination cases, but finding a drug company with the courage to invest in something new.

Bayer was founded in the German town of Barmen in 1863 – a former industrial metropolis that, interestingly, was also home to Friedrich Engels, co-founder of Marxist theory. Bayer's legend as a pharmaceutical giant was immortalised when they invented the original Aspirin in 1897. Chances are you already have some of their products in your bathroom, especially if your girlfriend takes the Dianette contraceptive.

They're also one of the few medical companies who looked into launching a male pill, but got cold feet. When I contacted them, a spokesperson admitted they considered the prospect, but 'discontinued the programme'. Hmmm. Was this due to concern over law suits from accidental pregnancies? Or is there simply more money to be made from keeping birth control a woman's domain? They refused to say. Even the Association of the British Pharmaceutical Industry, whose members supply 90 per cent of all NHS drugs, were tight-lipped.

Perhaps the stumbling block isn't willingness, but the practical difficulty of controlling millions of sperm as opposed to one egg. Likewise, the epic task of bringing a product to market isn't easy either. It goes a little something like this: after scientists make their initial lab discovery, bio-tech partners create a compound to prove it won't wreak havoc on the body's other cells. A prototype is then made for human drug testing, which is a three-stage, ten-year process conducted under strict medical supervision. Only then, if nobody dies or grows an extra limb, can it be considered for commercial use. At this point, a marketing plan must be devised to ensure the end product doesn't flop. And even then it's a risk.

'It's to do with maths,' says Dr Allan Pacey, Chair of the British Fertility Society and Senior Lecturer in Andrology at the University of Sheffield's Medical School. 'Both the methods and the market are already there. Ultimately, it's now about convincing the venture capitalists to step up, but it's extremely expensive.'

Fortunately, Pacey thinks Professor Smith stands a good chance because his approach has a unique selling point.

'All it will take is one of the smaller pharma companies [who are constantly looking for that competitive edge] to take the plunge,' he says. 'And because the latest developments centre around non-hormonal methods, it's much more likely to happen. Think of an independent record label launching a new act before a major buys them out.'

Weeks later, when back in London, I learn that male contraceptive research is still happening at Bayer – although on a small scale. Similarly, the World Health Organization is also continuing work in this field, as are America's National Institute for Health. In fact, the NIH are spending huge sums of government money on the discovery of new male methods.

Buoyed by this, I approach Pfizer – the world's largest drug-maker and producers of Viagra. I wonder if there's mileage in pitching the male contraceptive as a sex drug, but, once again, I'm greeted with radio silence. Perhaps, surrounded by all those little blue pills, everyone's too busy shagging to answer questions from journalists.

Undeterred, I track down Dr Peter Rost, Pfizer's former vice-president of marketing. Since his sensational departure from the company in 2005, which saw him fired after claiming that Pharmacia, a company Pfizer bought in 2003, illegally encouraged the sale of human growth hormones, he's reinvented himself as a bona fide media maverick. (US President Barack Obama's Chief of Staff, Rahm Emanuel, famously wanted to nominate him for a Guts of the Year award following his public swipe at his former employers.)

So, how would he sell it? 'It *would* be tough because

men don't have the fear factor of getting pregnant,' he says from his office in New Jersey. 'That's a very big marketing device with women. Instead, a better approach would be to imply that only the bravest men would take it. This isn't necessarily true,' he adds. 'But it taps into their psychology. Ultimately, echoing the control message of the 1960s would also work because men have never really had that – yet they want it.'

Whether a pharmaceutical giant would give it to them is another story, he adds. 'Yes, men would be very cautious about taking such a drug at first – because it's tinkering with their virility, albeit temporarily – but not nearly as much as the companies who are too scared to supply it.'

This isn't a lone theory. In an interview with *The Independent*, legendary Austrian-American scientist Carl Djerassi, the guy known as the father of the pill, voiced his own doubts on a male equivalent becoming a reality – because men don't demand it. 'This has nothing to do with science; we know exactly how to develop [the male pill], but there's not a single pharmaceutical company who will touch it – for economic and socio-political, rather than scientific, reasons.' he said. 'Their focus is on diseases of a geriatric population: diabetes, obesity, cardiovascular, Alzheimer's. Male contraception is nothing compared with an anti-obesity drug.'

Ironically, before his pill became commonplace in

1960s America, Djerassi's first marriage ended in divorce because he got a lover pregnant – after the condom broke. This fact, the idea that it could happen to the very man who created the solution, is a telling sign. If it can happen to him, it can happen to any one of us.

Days later, I find one of Peter Rost's books, *The Whistleblower: Confessions of a Healthcare Hitman*, in a charity shop. It's a shocking exposé of the medicine industry. Fascinated, I find a quiet corner in my local pub and read it within hours. As I leave, I nip to the bathroom. There, I see a condom machine. Rusty, empty and defaced with graffiti, it looks pathetic. Here is man's only real contraceptive choice – unavailable.

An old, dog-eared piece of paper with the words OUT OF ORDER! is sellotaped across it. My sentiments exactly, I think.

IN THE NAME OF
THE FATHER

THE SIGN ON THE SECURITY gate of Guy Harrison's West Sussex farm reads: 'Every breath you take, every step you make, I'll be watching you – The Police: you're on CCTV.'

Anti-establishment messages like this aren't a typical sight in the rolling acres of Ashurst, a sleepy village in the middle-class town of Horsham – especially from the likes of James Blunt's brother-in-law, whom you might expect to be a model citizen having posh pop peerage in the family – but it's a fitting nod to his cynicism for the powers that be.

Ten years ago, Guy was arrested under the Terrorism Act when he stormed the Houses of Parliament in 2004 and sensationally flour-bombed Tony Blair during Prime Minister's Questions. Detained and charged under Section Five of the Public Order Act, he faced two decades in a maximum-security prison and a lifetime of surveillance, but he wasn't a suicide bomber, a religious fanatic or even a Greenpeace activist. Nor was he protesting sexed-up dossiers and the Iraq War.

He was far more controversial than that: he was a father.

A self-made businessman, the 46-year-old is quite the unlikely anarchist. Born and raised in Guildford, he grew up on a farm next to the Surrey/Sussex border. He was an average student at local school St John's, where his most rebellious act was turning up one day on his father's tractor. He went on to become an estate agent in London, where his career took off – which is appropriate given that he famously met his wife, Emily, when James 'sold' his sister on eBay to whoever could get her to a funeral in Ireland amid an air traffic strike. Guy triumphed and used his private helicopter, which he'd bought 'for fun' from the Belgian military months earlier, to seal the deal. As you do.

Yet, as far as gestures go, this is pretty tame compared to the epic effort he made to see his first daughter, Isabella – the surprise product of a 'toxic' relationship which ended in 2001.

Take note, gentlemen.

'Oh, the stupidity of being a young man,' he jokes, deadpan.

> I'd been travelling around the world on the hundredth time we'd broken up. She'd written to me in Australia saying she had cervical cancer and was devastated, so I paid for her to have private healthcare. When I returned home we briefly reconciled and she immediately got pregnant. Little did I know I'd loaded the gun that would shoot me. It was only at the scan when the doctor let slip she'd had fertility treatment with the money – and there was no cancer, ever. It was the first of many traps.

Nine months later, Guy – less carefree man about town, more tasered single dad – graciously offered his ex and her new boyfriend £25,000 to fund a deposit on a home. They accepted, of course, but the Child Support Agency quickly ruled the generous sum was a 'gift' and could not be considered financial support for the baby, even though it was accompanied by a legal contract which described it so. The upshot? Guy was swiftly relieved of an additional £400 every month for eighteen years, totalling more than £100,000.

That's expensive sex.

Things went from bad to worse when his ex, who shall remain nameless, had two more children with her new boyfriend, which rendered Guy an immediate imperfection on their family portrait. Despite his best efforts to remain in the picture, including three court rulings that assured Sunday custody every other weekend – what a privilege! – she rewrote genetic history and dwindled his access to nothing: a christening took place without him, phone calls went unanswered and long-standing plans were suddenly scuppered at the last minute, never to be rescheduled. His money was welcome, but he wasn't.

The last time he saw his daughter was in a grey, lifeless supervision centre in Oxford, where he was forbidden from even taking her to the bathroom. That was fourteen years ago.

Caught in a pincer movement, he quickly built a legal case with a pricey City lawyer, hoping that if he kept calm, played by the rules and threw money at the problem, British justice would surely prevail. Sadly, in the words of The Clash, he fought the law and the law won. Having spent £50,000 on thirty-eight court appearances, his role was effectively erased by the state. His final, make-or-break battle took place on the same day two American Airlines planes crashed into New York's Twin Towers.

'That was my own personal 9/11,' he says.

> My ex was very well researched and played the system brilliantly. She knew a judge wouldn't jail her because she's a mother. They never do. Instead, he implemented a random two-year 'cooling-off period' because she was – in his words – 'implacably hostile'. It meant she could edit me from my daughter's life and I wouldn't be allowed to complain. There would be no threat of jail for her – even though she'd already disregarded existing court orders, no appeal, no intervention and absolutely no contact, during which time she could easily move away and start a new life. It was like state-sanctioned kidnapping.

Unsurprisingly, having exhausted all of his options, the months that followed were dominated with suicidal depression in what Guy calls 'a living bereavement'. When I gingerly ask him to describe his lowest point, aware that the wound is still raw, he pauses – but not to think. He already knows the answer. Rather, choked on emotion, he is trying not to break down in front of me.

'I had a rifle in my mouth,' he says, lowly. 'It was a very, very dark time.'

Thankfully, in a do-or-die decision, he channelled his energy into one of the few sympathetic groups for dis-enfranchised dads: Fathers 4 Justice – the controversial men-in-tights organisation who scale buildings as super-heroes to change sexist family law. There, he spent four years fielding calls from thousands of men who, like him, never thought it would happen to them. Yet, here they were: navigating the same soul-destroying, dead-end, bullshit process with desperate pleas for help falling on deaf ears.

'Every six weeks there would be a suicide and we'd scrub their name off the list,' he throws in, casually. 'That's how normalised the desperation was. Men were literally dying to see their own children.'

But, despite the trauma, his work became a strange form of by-proxy therapy. Fortified by it, and with noth-ing left to lose, he became stronger. Politically motivated. Happy to risk life and limb on stunts which demanded attention as well as answers. Which is how he found himself in Parliament, stood before our country's (then) most powerful person, holding a condom filled – rather cheekily – with 'self-raising' flour. Credit where credit's due: at least he had a sense of humour about it.

The rest, as they say, is history.

A decade on, as we take a seat in his immaculate living room – littered with pictures of his children with Emily, one-year-old Lola and Hugh, three – he vividly describes his arrest and the hours that followed at Paddington Green police station: a place typically reserved for suspected terrorists, not eager fathers. There were the good cop/bad cop cross-examinations which took place every three hours – even throughout the night, the fetid stench of the squalid cell and the gritty reality that, pretty often, justice miscarries when you're a bloke. Even if your motivation is good.

'I'd be rubbish in a Jack Bauer situation,' he admits with a wry smile.

> They could break me with Morris dancers, but the police still made me feel like I was in Guantanamo Bay. I confidently thought I'd be out in twenty-four hours, but they took great delight in telling me I'd be held without charge for fourteen days and, if convicted, imprisoned for up to twenty-one years. As far as they were concerned I'd breached Her Majesty's Parliament and was up there with Abu Hamza.

I can't help but laugh. As he pushes a well-curated biscuit barrel under my nose and serves tea in a china cup, it's clear that this well-spoken, charming man – a gentleman and a gentle man, dressed in foppish chinos and a polo club T-shirt – is hardly a danger to national security. Christ, he even wrote to Downing Street and offered to pay Blair's dry-cleaning bill following their tête-à-tête (who, in turn, replied saying he was very sympathetic to the cause, but couldn't be seen to accept the offer in case it upset his Blair Babes – ta very much).

Despite this, five days on trial in Southwark Crown Court followed, as did five solid years of *Homeland*-style surveillance which was itself a daily white-knuckle ride. 'Nobody saw the aftermath of the arrest once the TV cameras disappeared,' he adds.

> The trial was psychologically gruelling, truly terrifying, and the threat of a custodial sentence was absolutely real. I endured three tax investigations, was forced to shut businesses in America and Australia, couldn't travel abroad and had my house bugged. At one point eight policemen stormed the front door and searched my property for traces of ricin, which didn't even exist. Hilariously, I had to give them the pin code for the gate because they couldn't get past it. In hindsight, the only funny thing about it was that, quite often, the police were utterly fucking stupid.

Hence the sign.

Even Emily, who, at a guess, is probably about as bellicose as Kate Middleton, was arrested as the milieu unfolded. A fact that's hard to comprehend when you meet her because she's so poised, respectful and well-mannered. But as she sits there recanting the tale – beautiful, clever, calm and WASPy – I realise that her Blunt DNA is startlingly evident. She is her famous brother liquidised, shaken up and poured into female form. Meanwhile, the real criminal, Isabella's mother, escaped justice because of her own physical attributes: specifically, her gender. A reality which is less the exception, more the rule when it comes to family breakdown.

'It all depends on whether fathers are listed on the birth certificate,' says solicitor Vanessa Lloyd-Platt.

> That technically determines parental responsibility, but yes, mothers usually get custody. Typically, men are fed into the system – told to write letters, get a lawyer and wait for a court date – but this can take months, even years. In that time the ex-wives can have new boyfriends, new houses, new names.
>
> Incongruously, time is of the essence for fathers but the system deliberately facilitates against anything moving quickly. Of course, the longer it goes on, the harder it is for them to re-establish contact with an estranged child. The latest version of the court system, which only

launched in April 2014, is already in chaos. I've seen cases listed for a year that are suddenly cancelled the night before because there aren't enough judges. They were all retired off with their pensions at the same time legal funding got cut, so the system is completely clogged up with cases. Fighting for access is hard enough, but now most men can't even get into court to start.

It wasn't always this way. In the 1800s men typically got custody of their children, but not as a result of naked privilege. They were solely financially responsible for them, too. Yes, they got the children, but they also got the bill. Benefits Britain didn't exist.

Now, 200 years on, women get the kids, but men still get the bill. Sometimes men even pay for children that aren't theirs. The Child Support Agency have roughly 500 cases of paternity fraud per year – and they're just the ones we know about. According to a YouGov study, 1.2 million British men doubt their parentage.

The recent case of Steven Carter is not unusual: the CSA deducted £50,000 from his accounts between 2007 and 2014 – even though a DNA test later proved the child in question wasn't his. They acknowledged this, but the Department of Work and Pensions still won't refund him because the 'child' is now twenty-two – thus an adult – so the case is closed. Then there's Mark Webb, who raised his 'daughter' for seventeen years only to discover they were no relation. When he sued his ex-wife for compensation, both county and appeal court judges denied his damages claim, brushing it off as a man's obligation.

To this day no British woman has ever been convicted of paternity fraud.

This set-up is no accident. Since Harriet Harman and her pals entered politics, the laws which govern family life have been re-jigged to put women on top – and men on the back foot. Together, they decided families weren't society's natural, balanced building block, but a cunning plot to oppress mothers whilst placing men in undeserving positions of power (when, actually, men were breaking their backs in jobs they hated just to keep everything ticking over). To avenge this, they squeezed men from the home and hit them where it hurts: the heart.

Don't believe me? The Children Act 1989 specifically declares: 'The rule of law that a father is the natural guardian of his legitimate child is abolished.'

A year later, a 1990 report by the Institute for Public Policy Research called 'The Family Way' saw Harriet personally declare: 'It cannot be assumed that men are bound to be an asset to family life or that the presence of fathers in families is necessarily a means to social cohesion.' Meanwhile, American feminist Linda Gordon ruled: 'The nuclear family must be destroyed … whatever its ultimate meaning.'

Even now, the Children and Families Bill doesn't mention the word 'father' once. Not once.

Fast-forward to the present day and Isabella is one of four million children who are products of this. On the bright side, at least Guy's in good company: Sir Bob Geldof was one of the first high-profile men to address the issue after losing access to his daughters Peaches, Pixie and Fifi when Paula Yates left him back in 1995. This should alarm even the most successful man, because, if raising millions to ease Ethiopian famine through Live Aid doesn't render you decent father material, the rest of us are – to be frank – fucked.

When I met him at a party in west London some time later, he confessed that fighting the system nearly bankrupted him. 'It was beyond expensive,' he told me.

> I had to borrow money and was close to losing it all. In the end my circumstances changed naturally, but it could've been very different. Men still spend thousands of pounds getting court orders that aren't worth the paper they're written on. The whole system is disgusting. I remember a court clerk at my trial telling me: 'Whatever you do, don't say you love your children. Family courts consider men who articulate this as extreme.' It was madness.

Hollywood actor Jason Patric, who's best known for *The Lost Boys* and *Sleepers*, is locked in a similar battle. He and his ex, Danielle Schreiber, dated for ten years before they split, proving that even the most promising relationship can hit the skids – and, when it does, women can become pawn stars. No, not porn stars – but pawn stars, you know: the type of mother who uses her child as a weapon to enact revenge for a broken heart. Like a pawn in a game. Classy work, ladies.

He too ended up in court trying to see his own son, who lives just ten minutes away from him in LA. In a bid to highlight his situation, he set up a site called Stand Up For Gus, where he detailed the jaw-dropping twists and turns of the story. Unimpressed, she tried to censor it with a gagging order, but he fought back and won – like any decent lad should. Mark Wahlberg, Chris Rock, Chris Evans, Mel Gibson and *Mad Men*'s Jon Hamm all backed the cause in a penalty wall of Men United, which is exactly what we need more of, because these stories aren't rare. They're not even few and far between. They happen all over the world, constantly.

According to the Office for National Statistics, one in three youngsters now have no access to their father – which equates to four million children in the UK.

Reassuringly, there's been some very creative resistance. If the fathers' rights movement was once in its Modigliani phase – one of reflection, sadness and alienation – it's now surely in its Rothko era: bold, modern and surreal. In 2013, 58-year-old Paul Douglas Manning was arrested at London's National Gallery for affixing a photograph of his son to the canvas of John Constable's master-piece *The Hay Wain*. This followed Tim Haries' arrest for spraying the word 'Help' on a Ralph Heimans por-trait of the Queen in Westminster Abbey. Not because they're common vandals, but because they're crying for help. Desperate times call for desperate measures and all that. They had to break the law to shake the law, which – quite frankly – is the bigger criminal offence. See, if the legal process actually enforced men's civic rights as they're paid huge sums to do, there'd be no need for peaceful protests.

Either way, all this is further proof that parenthood is rarely a bronco worth backing. In fact, for many men it's an old nag that needs shooting. The odds of it crossing the line are atrocious. I doubt William Hill would even take bets on it. Not least because, despite stellar efforts from some really great men and women, the law seems to have remained exactly the same as it was ten, twenty, thirty years ago. Nothing has changed. Right?

'If you'd asked me that last year I would've agreed,' says Dr Craig Pickering from charity Families Need Fathers.

> But the Children and Families Act 2014 says, for the first
> time in English law, that both parents should be involved
> in a child's life after a divorce. Trouble is, its effectiveness
> depends on what the judges make of it. And it wouldn't
> be the first time they came up with their own bizarre
> interpretation of something straight-forward – but at
> least there's hope.

When I ask him how this will be possible when court
orders have less traction than England at a World Cup, he
offers a plausible solution. 'We need similar sanctions to
those who won't pay child support: passports and driving
licences confiscated. These things don't affect the child,
but they inconvenience the parent directly. The current
government consulted on this and there was quite some
optimism, but they stopped mid-way through. We don't
know why.'

Oh.

I put this to Edward Timpson MP, Minister for Children and Families, who's the man in charge. My message
gets passed to somebody else, who passes it onto somebody else, who passes it onto somebody else. Eventually,
the Ministry of Justice tells me: 'The consultation con-
cluded that we should not introduce further punitive
enforcement elements. There are already punishments
available.' Hmm. Perhaps somebody needs to tell them

they don't *actually* work. Not for fathers or children. The same children who – if they're lucky – are being raised by random men, whose kids are being raised by other men, whose kids are being raised by other men.

Considering the annual cost of family breakdown is reportedly £44 billion – yep, that's more than the defence budget – you'd think curing fatherlessness would be a priority for a country haemorrhaging money, but it isn't. Instead, everybody's petrified of inadvertently apportioning blame to single mothers – *even though it's not about them*. Only recently, in a bid to woo the female vote – which is a golden ticket when it comes to the ballot box – David Cameron said deadbeat dads 'should be looked at like drink drivers', yet said nothing about the mothers who deliberately steer them off the road. Here we had the head of British government telling men to raise children properly, yet offering a law that actively keeps children and fathers apart as the solution.

Perhaps he should try going through the system to see his children if Sam Cam shacks up with Ed Balls and poisons them against him. It'd be a bit like the BBC's *Back to the Floor*, except useful.

Then again, this isn't ignorance – he doesn't *want* to address it. Rather than face reality, annoy a few female MPs and co-ordinate with Fathers 4 Justice to improve the law, he'd prefer to kiss politically correct ass. To date, despite the epidemic of fatherlessness, F4J have always been excluded from state committee meetings on shared parenting, irrespective of the fact that they're the UK's biggest authority on the matter.

Admittedly, thousands of years of war and violence haven't done us any favours. Men have long been considered aggressors and threats to the safety of children, rightly or wrongly, but let's be honest: women aren't perfect parents either. Fucking up is a human trait, not a male defect. In fact, in the last few years, the highest-profile culprits of child abuse have been mothers. There's the infamous Karen Matthews, Amanda Hutton – whose son's mummified body was found two years after he died – and, of course, Baby P's Tracey Connelly.

'There is absolutely *no* magic ingredient women have when it comes to being parents,' says Adrienne Burgess from the Fatherhood Institute.

> Both genders know nothing when their babies are first born. Everybody's cack-handed. It's something a person learns on the job and, as they do, their bodies attune. Studies prove that becoming a father happens in your body, just as it does with women. A man's hormonal balance actually changes as he holds a baby.

> Men are equally innately hard-wired to care for chil-
> dren. The only difference is that the rest of the world
> think they're dangerous, uninterested and lacking skills
> which mothers are born with. That is a total myth. Sadly,
> the health system – including midwives – and the media
> treat fathers like a joke.

Ah, yes – the media. Off the top of my head I can cite
Men Behaving Badly, *Shameless*, *Last of the Summer Wine*,
The Simpsons, *Peppa Pig*, *Two and a Half Men*, *Everybody
Loves Raymond* and *Friends* as examples, plus, for the sake
of a classic childhood reference, *Three Men and a Baby*,
which, BTW, was the highest-grossing box office hit of
1987. Oh, how we laughed at those docile dads.

Getting her political priorities mixed up, actress Helen
Mirren chided 007 director Sam Mendes at the Empire
awards for having the audacity to list his role models as
Paul Thomas Anderson, François Truffaut, Martin Scorsese
and Ingmar Bergman. The problem? They were all blokes.
This, she said, was sexist. Male role models are bad unless
accompanied by oestrogen. Yet she says nothing about the
likes of Kate Winslet, Sam's ex-wife, who famously told
Vogue magazine: 'None of this 50/50 time with the mums
and dads – my children live with me; that is it.'

Then there's Halle Berry, who tried to take her daughter away from her father, Gabriel Aubry, by relocating to

France – relocation, relocation, relocation being a common tactic in this situation. Yet, it was she who chose to have a child with him in the first place. She who made all the big decisions about whether to continue with the pregnancy. She who had opportunities to opt out at any time. He didn't. Meanwhile, single-parent organisations like Gingerbread – supported by children's author J. K. Rowling of all people – casually dismiss studies which suggest a lack of male role models at home increases the likelihood of crime and mental illness.

This is despite a study conducted by Oxford University which followed nearly 20,000 children from 1958 and found those with a father were far less likely to break the law or suffer from psychological issues. Young boys with involved fathers also performed better at school. Meanwhile, Dr Paul Ramchandani of Imperial College London found that 'disengaged and remote father–child interactions as early as the third month of life' predict behaviour problems in children when they are older.

Granted, this isn't conclusive, of course. But, even if this was just an elaborate hoax to make people feel sorry for fathers, surely we could all agree that needlessly removing men from families would at least make *some* boys feel like shit *some* of the time? The logic is simple – not having a father leaves a hole in the soul. A void that kids frequently fill with drugs, alcohol or intimacy. This might not sit well in the feminist family framework, but sometimes the truth is a bitch.

In 2012 British substance misuse charity Addaction published a report that proved father deficit to be absolutely real – causing anger, self-loathing, addiction and identity issues. Specifically, it saw young men compensate with a 'counterfeit masculinity' of strength, anger and violence – often combined with sexual prowess. Meanwhile, young women 'act out a skewed version of femininity which prioritises the use of sex and relationships with men above all else'.

Cruelly, this creates the cycle all over again because boys of fifteen often jump into bed with a girl without a nagging, ball-tightening paranoia that she'll get pregnant. And here's the bit nobody else will admit: loads of girls *do* want to get pregnant. They get a free house, FFS! I'd get pregnant for a free house!

The Trust for the Study of Adolescence recently proved that scores of teenage girls are *deliberately* becoming young mothers as a career move because, with both the state and father contributing, it offers more guaranteed security than a job. Even thirteen-year-old girls admitted this, which might explain why Britain has the highest teenage pregnancy rate in Europe, at an annual governmental cost of nearly £63 million.

Obviously, this doesn't mean that women are to blame

for manipulating the system because they're female. They do so because they can. The set-up encourages them to take advantage, like journalists at a free bar. Likewise, if men held all the aces, we'd do the same. Which is why the solution must be gender-neutral.

Perhaps if law-makers continue to ignore this they should offer some other alternatives. Maybe men could be allowed to have a financial abortion from a child they didn't pre-consent to. In a specified time period – say, legal abortion guidelines – men could be allowed to formally relinquish all monetary obligations, rights and responsibilities if duped into daddydom. The woman still wants to proceed? Fine, that's her choice. But not on his salary.

Controversial? Yes. But overnight we'd see fewer acts of conception by deception. I once knew a girl who was so desperate to have a baby she went on dating sites to fuck men – but only after piercing their condoms with a pin. She now has a two-year-old child and the father, who was reduced to the role of donor and walking cash-point, barely gets a look-in (but pays hundreds every month).

Then there are those who sleep with minors, get pregnant and demand child support FROM A CHILD. In 1993 a thirteen-year-old Kansas boy impregnated his seventeen-year-old babysitter, but the Supreme Court ruled that he was liable for maintenance. Apparently, the financial aid was for the resulting baby, not the rapist, so that's OK.

A similar case is County of San Luis Obispo v. Nathaniel J. in California, which saw a 34-year-old woman seduce a fifteen-year-old boy, get pregnant and demand child support. The courts upheld her claim, which essentially ruled that a male victim of statutory rape should be forced into financial slavery if a baby results from the crime.

Thankfully, and perhaps most compellingly, one of the people pushing hardest for change is herself a woman – Nadine O'Connor is the campaign director at Fathers 4 Justice. I know what you're thinking: why on earth would a woman want that gig? After all, no matter how liberated women have become in recent years, the partnership remains an unlikely one.

It turns out she had her own personal experience of what men frequently endure in family law courts. The mother of two went through her own custody battle with her ex-partner, which clocked up twenty-five judges, seventy hearings, fifty-four criminal allegations, forty-five court orders and over £120,000 in legal bills.

'I went to the first F4J meeting with my dad,' she says.

> If they'd been plotting to take power away from mothers then, obviously, I wouldn't have stayed. But they

simply ask to be given the same rights as them. To this day, what most people fail to realise is that the current law can disenfranchise grandparents, stepmothers and siblings too – not just men. I spend much of my working day with women who can't see loved ones through no fault of their own.

This is something Guy's wife, Emily, can surely relate to. She's never met her stepdaughter and, as a result, has become her own surprise advocate for the cause. This wasn't the expected fate for a woman of her pedigree.

'I was very much a lady of the establishment,' she explains.

My father was senior in the army [he ran a famous British Army base near the Hampshire village of Middle Wallop] and I always believed good prevailed. I trusted that people in positions of power would do the right thing. I had faith in the system. But, without a shadow of a doubt, there is bias and corruption – I saw it myself in Guy's case. It shattered my innocence.

This rude awakening came at the same time her chart-topping brother announced his engagement to long-term girlfriend Sofia Wellesley, the granddaughter of the Duke of Wellington.

'It's important to get the right girl and, as a man, to be aware of the law,' Guy adds.

> That is what I've told James, but it applies to everyone. You can't be happy when you've had your child taken away and, currently, the law hates fathers. If they were ever to have children and separate, he would be powerless – despite his wealth. Most men in this country have no idea what they're up against because it plays out in secret courts. They don't stand a chance if it all goes wrong.

Fortunately, although his name might sound like Cockney rhyming slang, the 'You're Beautiful' singer is anything but a fool. He's accustomed to strength in adversity no matter what happens. Not just in Kosovo, where he once served, but somewhere much scarier: online. When one woman famously trolled him on Twitter saying: 'I have this dire need to listen to James Blunt when I'm menstruating,' he replied: 'Useful feedback. I'll pass this on to my marketing team.' When someone else asked: 'Who is a bigger twat: James Blunt or Robin Thicke?' he said: 'Me! Me! Pick me!' Then, when another posted: 'Jesus Christ, James Blunt's got a new album out. Is there anything else that can go wrong?' he deadpanned: 'Yes. He could start tweeting you.'

Now that's having the last laugh.

Hopefully, Guy might get his one day, too – although, when we catch up three months after our initial meeting, I realise that it's not likely to happen any time soon.

'We've just received news that Isabella's been moved to Australia – conveniently, right before her eighteenth birthday,' he says, gutted. 'The entire family have emigrated for good. Just like that, even though my ex isn't legally allowed to relocate without informing me first, but since when did rules matter? All that counts is that I keep paying up. The nightmare just never ends.'

Thrown, I offer some optimism, but it falls spectacularly short. Nothing I can do or say could possibly make a difference because, ultimately, nothing ever *does* make a difference. Not the law, not the courts, not even the Prime Minister when he's confronted in Parliament.

It all colludes to mark the start of an awkward silence that nothing can fill.

Then, something happens. 'Oh, by the way, did I ever tell you that James's fiancée works for Tony's wife, Cherie Booth?' he chips in, brighter. 'That'll be a bloody interesting wedding. Let's hope we're on the same table.'

We both force a laugh and swallow our frustrations. It's only weeks later, when I'm having a tour of the Houses of Parliament – with, bizarrely, Sir Ian McKellen – that I see a glass panel separating the public gallery from the debating chamber.

'This was put in after a man threw purple flour at Tony Blair – and scored an impressive hit!' the guide says, unaware of my connection. 'Poor bloke, just wanted to see his daughter – but clearly didn't realise that once his ex made her mind up, that was it. Not even the PM could change that.'

It's only then that it hits me, hard.

It's not politicians, world leaders or judges who stop fathers seeing their children. Nor is it the creaking family law courts. The unpalatable truth, which goes against our instinctive values as protectors, is that it's women.

Until we acknowledge this fact head-on – and end the romantic myth around matriarchs – it'll remain the mother of every father's inequality.

CIRCUMCISION: THE FIRST CUT IS THE DEEPEST

WHEN A LEOPARD-PRINT-CLAD Rod Stewart sang Cat Stevens's classic 'The First Cut Is the Deepest' back in 1977, it was a simple reference to the broken-hearted, but listen to it now and, thirty years on, it seems the raspy rocker may have had an early insight into where the politics of the penis would eventually end up. Because those famous lyrics – 'She's taken almost all that I've got / but if you want I'll try to love again' – could easily be lifted and superimposed onto a more serious, cutting-edge issue for lads and dads. A practice which fuses religion with history and – more importantly – sharp knives with penises. A combination that should never meet in the same sentence, never mind real life. Yet, every year, hordes of baby boys endure exactly that: they have a blade taken to their foreskin within days of being born – some in the name of religion, some for lazy tradition, others for a parent's vanity.

Whatever the reason, let's be clear: it was highly appropriate when comedians Penn and Teller trashed it in their Showtime series *Bullshit!* But allow me to elaborate.

According to statistics from the National Center for Disease Control, more than a million unnecessary circumcisions are performed in the US alone every year. That's one every thirty seconds or, by Premier League standards, Anfield Stadium filled twenty-five times. Here in the UK the number of modified kids is thought to be considerably fewer, around 20 per cent of British boys, but that's still a teary-eyed tally of thousands.

The very first circumcision is thought to have happened in Egypt centuries ago and, since then, has been performed for religious reasons in Jewish and Muslim communities across the Middle East. But it only became popular in the West during the late nineteenth century when Victorian killjoys wanted to discourage people from masturbating. No, seriously.

Not to put you off your breakfast, but one of the biggest advocates of this was Michigan physician Dr John Harvey Kellogg – yep, the man behind your corn flakes. A medical practitioner and businessman, he also doubled as a sex prude who wouldn't consummate his marriage, slept in a separate room to his wife and adopted each of their children (rather than producing them the fun way). Not content with his own monastic life, he wanted to discourage everybody else from pleasure too, so suggested two ways of making this happen: young girls should receive a dab of carbolic acid to the clitoris, which would burn and produce numb scar tissue, whilst boys should have the hoods of their foreskins cut off.

Both methods were designed with one specific, leg-crossing aim: to tame lust in the young. This, they thought, would get people out of the bedroom and into the workforce, creating a wholesome, healthy, wealthy society that feared intimacy as much as it did God.

Fortunately, the former didn't catch on – but the latter did. In modern Twitter terminology we'd say it started trending, but – decades on – long after Kellogg died, it remains the biggest legacy from the Victorian vault of sexual eccentricities. Yet, because it happens to boys, who must surely deserve it for simply being boys, countless babies are still being lined up to have their tips snipped in what is, quite literally, a bloody liberty.

Dr John Warren was one of them. A retired doctor who worked at the Alexandra Hospital in Harlow, his experience formed a full revolution of opinion over forty years, going from cuttee to cutter to campaigner. He was so hacked off – pardon the pun – that he went on to form Britain's first anti-circumcision organisation, Norm UK, which tells institutions like the General Medical Council to cut it out, not off. Their big break came when Jeremy Paxman invited him onto *Newsnight* and sided with them over a notoriously staunch rabbi, declaring that foreskin removal was indeed a sexist slice of life, not a symbol of faith.

'There were three stages in becoming an intactivist,' he tells me.

> When I was four years old I had a bath with my brother and noticed his penis was different. When I asked why, my mother said I'd had an operation that my father hadn't approved of, but he died in war so she went ahead with it anyway.
>
> Years later I took up medicine like all the other men in my family. One day in surgical training they wheeled

a seven-year-old boy into theatre and told me to circumcise him, so I did. This was the first time I could unravel a foreskin and actually appreciate the amount of tissue there was – and, believe me, there was a *lot*. Not many men get to see this, but it was my second epiphany because the skin wasn't diseased in any way, yet I still had to remove it. I suffered many sleepless nights over that decision and never did another circumcision again.

But it was only later in life that John, now seventy-one, experienced the reality of what circumcision meant in his own sex life. 'I was getting middle-aged and I had very little feeling in my penis,' he confesses, frankly.

I didn't really know what was happening down there. I'd go through the motions but not feel very much. The head had no sensation. At first I assumed everybody was like this, then, of course, I joined the dots. I realised it was because I had no foreskin. It was a delayed reaction, but I was devastated.

Scientifically, what he describes is the helmet of a healthy penis keratinising, which means it hardens like a callus in the absence of a nourishing foreskin. Something that happens in varying degrees to all circumcised men.

Despite this, most people – especially new parents

– have no idea what the procedure does, yet they go ahead with it anyway, which is surprising given that boy-cutting doesn't have a great track record. Perhaps most famously, it caused the death of David Reimer, whose tragic tale is the ultimate cock cover-up and was the first case to raise a question mark over the practice in the '70s.

Born Bruce Reimer in Winnipeg, Canada, 1965, he was raised female after a botched circumcision totally destroyed his penis in a tragic, but surprisingly common, complication.

When he was just six months old, doctors used a method called cauterisation – the medical equivalent of ridding skin with a flambé torch – to remove the hood of his foreskin, but a trigger-happy practitioner went too far and damaged the entire organ. Panicked, doctors convinced his devastated parents to brush the complication under the carpet by raising him female with a combination of drugs, dresses and trendy social conditioning that said gender was learned, not embedded in DNA.

At twenty-two months old he underwent an orchidectomy, which means his testes were forcibly removed, then – as if that wasn't bad enough – he had to answer to the name of Brenda.

From here he urinated through a hole in his abdomen whilst taking oestrogen shots to induce breast growth, never knowing he was actually a little boy starring in his own equivalent of *The Truman Show*. Some time later he was scheduled to have a makeshift vagina built into his groin, but this was shelved when – at thirteen – he started battling suicidal depression. He diagnosed himself with gender identity crisis, which wasn't far off the mark. The only difference being that his version was man-made.

In 1980, when he was fourteen, Reimer's parents eventually came clean when they realised no amount of social steering could rewrite the genetic truth that he was male, not female. Nature 1, gender politics 0.

Reimer instantly resumed his male persona and underwent gruelling re-reassignment surgery to correct the damage, including a double mastectomy, testosterone injections and two phalloplasty operations, which saw doctors try to make a replica 'penis' with skin grafts. Eventually, in his twenties, he married and became a stepfather to three children, but when his wife left him in 2004, he shot himself in the head with a sawn-off shotgun, capping an utterly so-called life. He was just thirty-eight.

Since then, people haven't just started questioning boy-cutting, but also the religion that promotes it – which is perhaps its trickiest sticking point. After all, nobody wants to offend or, worse, be seen as anti-Semitic. But in an age of Richard Dawkins and popular atheism, the debate isn't quite so off-limits as it once was. For Ron Goldman from the American organisation Jews Against

Circumcision, such fear of offending is getting in the way of a bigger issue.

'We are a group of educated and enlightened Jews who realise that the primitive practice of genital cutting has no place in modern Judaism,' he says. 'And we should know. Jews are some of the smartest people in the world,' he jokes. 'We hold a third of Nobel Peace Prizes, which means we're smart enough to understand that mutilating a little boy's penis is not an acceptable practice in modern times. Besides, God did not mandate circumcision. In the original version of the Torah, the book of J, it's not even mentioned.'

Another US campaign group, Beyond the Bris, are equally vocal. A grassroots anti-cutting site which steers fellow Jewish parents away from the procedure, it's run by mother-of-three Rebecca Wald, who's already kickstarted new thinking. 'Things are definitely changing, even in my average, everyday neighbourhood,' she says from the East Coast. 'The internet has helped spread a lot of information and people are finally waking up. When Jewish people themselves make this choice about something so traditional, it speaks volumes. We're a liberal bunch.' I tested this theory myself. When I called two of London's most prominent modern synagogues – the West London Synagogue and the Central Synagogue – neither of them had an issue with me bringing my fictitious, non-circumcised son to services. One of them even added: 'It's not like we're going to check.' Thank God for that. Not least because it means we're not anti-Semitic for wanting to stop our sons having their bodies modified at birth.

And there's even more good news. Although it's still in its infancy, the 'intactivist' movement, which is a genius bit of branding, has already seen procedure rates take a 10 per cent drop in popularity across the United States as knowledge – like flood water – finds a route past obstacles. Look at the stats: almost two-thirds of US boys in the late '70s were cut, but that percentage dropped to around 58 per cent in 2010.

It's official: times are changing.

San Francisco has been on the cusp of change for years, with everything from green issues to the technological boom. It's also the place that brought us Instagram and Twitter, so it's no coincidence that the City by the Bay was also one of the first places to try to ban circumcision in law. Just like Australia gets the first taste of New Year sun, San Francisco seems to be the same with new, progressive concepts. A formal motion to outlaw circumcision was filed and would've passed, but it was dropped from the Senate ballot by a senior High Court judge at the last minute. Still, it was a start – and one that sparked a chain reaction. A short time later there was a circumcision ban in Cologne, but Angela Merkel overturned it and now it appears Norway is about to implement a similar ruling.

Objectors aren't exclusive to the US though. There have also been mainstream, credible British equivalents. The late, great Christopher Hitchens was one of the few people who dared discuss this subject in public. There's a brilliant video online of him 'hitchslapping' a rabbi who claims 'My son cried more at his first haircut than his bris,' at which point Hitchens spins around and says:

> Actually, I don't find genital mutilation funny. The full removal of the foreskin is fantastically painful, leads to the dulling of the sexual relationship and can cause death. It is a blatant attempt to cripple the male organ of generation. What next – cutting the labia of little girls? What would you think of me if I said my daughter cried more at her first haircut than when I cut her clitoris off?

You could hear a pin drop in the auditorium.

But fair play to him. After all, a penis is just as valuable as a vagina – right? Well, so you'd like to think. Yet the debate around circumcision has already become gendered, meaning boys are expected to put up and shut up, whilst women demand an end to girl-cutting. And only girl-cutting, even though they're similar.

'Oh, there's absolutely a comparison,' says Rebecca Wald.

> There's a continuum of FGM [female genital mutilation] and the equivalent of male circumcision is definitely on there, whether people like it or not. Some forms of FGM are just a pin-prick, which is obviously still bad, but it's nowhere near as terrible as foreskin removal. The whole thing has become political. As a mother, I'm amazed that there are people dedicated to saving girls' genital integrity who couldn't care less about boys'. It's definitely a men's rights issue. One hundred per cent.

Interestingly, she also sees it as a woman's issue. 'Most of my audience are women,' she adds. 'Which is interesting, because it's a son's mother who hands him over to be operated on in the first place. Her boy is taken with her full consent, when – like a lioness – she should be opposing it. But where are the feminists?'

Good question. Currently, London's biggest free newspaper, the *Evening Standard*, is edited by Sarah Sands. She's made it her mission to put female circumcision on the map as an issue of misogyny, yet says nothing when the equivalent practice affects boys. In fact, she pretty much refuses to acknowledge it at all. When I met her at a party in Battersea Power Station for London's

most powerful 1,000 people, she'd given a speech introducing the night's entertainment – a woman who had
suffered female circumcision and, for the benefit of party
guests, was going to sing about it. In detail. But when I
approached Sands to ask if she could expand her paper's
standpoint to include boys, she shushed me.

I tried again, but was given a death stare. The difference, she said, was that, for girls, the procedure is
designed to affect sexual function, whilst for boys it
is simply a hygiene issue.

'That's bullshit,' says Jonathon Conte, a Californian
campaigner who's part of a radical new generation of
anti-cutting activists across the USA, peacefully protesting everywhere from paediatric conferences to the White
House.

> Regardless of the sex of the victim, a healthy individ-
> ual being restrained without their consent and having
> their genitals removed is a violation. In its purest form
> the removal of the prepuce, which is the same struc-
> ture anatomically in men and women, it's entirely an
> analogous procedure. Besides, we shouldn't be arguing
> about what's better or worse. It shouldn't be a compe-
> tition of suffering, everybody has the right to grow up
> with their whole body. As an adult if you want to have
> a body modification – a tattoo, a piercing, cosmetic

> surgery or circumcision – great, go for it, but children
> aren't property.

True. Both procedures remove functional tissue, cause extreme pain, permanently disfigure the genitals and forever damage the sexual response. And in most cultures where female circumcision is performed, male circumcision is also performed with equally dirty, blunt apparatus.

Bizarrely, whilst the intactivism movement does have support from both genders, there are countless women like Sands who want to keep it a feminist hot topic. When Lynne Featherstone MP – the Equalities Minister, FFS – waded into the FGM debate, she said: 'It's a practice that has been going on for 4,000 years and, without wishing to be crude about this, quite frankly if it was boys' willies that were being cut off without anaesthetic it wouldn't have lasted four minutes, let alone 4,000 years.'

Err, except it has – and still is.

Another charmer is *The Guardian*'s Tanya Gold. When the Council of Europe made a recommendation to ban the circumcision of girls *and* boys, she mused it was anti-Semitic and sexist, saying: in the 'legislative warmth and kind ideals was the Jew bomb; the revolting juxtaposition of female genital mutilation, which is always torture, and often murder, with ritual male circumcision, which is neither.'

Er, sorry – get your facts straight. In September 2012, a two-week-old infant died at a Brooklyn hospital after contracting herpes through a circumcision ritual called metzitzah b'peh, which involves the bleeding foreskin coming into contact with the mouth of the mohel, who sucks it dry. In November 2012, Manchester Crown Court heard how a four-week-old boy bled to death after a DIY home circumcision went wrong. Nurse Grace Adeleye was paid £100 to carry out the procedure, using only scissors, forceps and olive oil, at the family home in Chadderton. Adeleye was later found guilty of manslaughter by gross negligence. Chillingly, her defence recounted that thousands of boys are routinely circumcised in this way in Nigeria, as if that's somehow a mitigating circumstance.

Likewise, Californian baby Brayden Tyler Frazier died in 2013. The newborn child, who was only a few days old, suffered serious complications as a result of the procedure and died from his injuries on 8 March. Ironically, his death coincided with International Women's Day, which is designed to effect positive change between the sexes. Oh, the irony.

Yet, as a nation, we still have our priorities all wrong. Shop mannequins are being made to look fatter so women don't feel bad for eating three KitKat Chunkys during *The X Factor*, but millions of boys are still suffering the indignity of having their dicks diced. What the hell is going on?

Perhaps the reason people are so mind-numbingly stupid when it comes to this issue is because the words we use to describe it have lost their shock value. Maybe our current vocabulary isn't controversial enough; our arguments have become dulled and blunt with overuse – unlike the surgical knives used. They are no longer sufficiently serrated or hard-hitting to describe the grimness of it all. So what do we call it? Male genital mutilation? Son-slashing? Cock-crippling? Maybe words aren't enough, full stop. Perhaps what people really need is to see raw images of raw penises on babies. Gruesome shots of exactly what happens when a boy is strapped down, has his perfectly fine and functioning foreskin clamped then cut, in an often unregulated practice.

One of the weakest pro-arguments people present is that young boys should 'look like their dad'. But, hang on, how often do we see our father's penis? It's not like you go to a family party and distant relatives look down your trousers and say, 'Ah, you're the spitting image of your dad!'

Then there's the hygiene excuse. The World Health Organization says circumcised boys help reduce the risk of heterosexually acquired HIV infection by 60 per cent. But, last time I checked, baby boys weren't having sex.

And when the time comes there's always our friends at Durex. Besides, if circumcision prevented HIV so much, why is America still a nation with high transmission rates? In 2011, 49,273 people were diagnosed with HIV in the United States. In that same year, more than 32,000 people had full-blown AIDS.

WHICH CLEARLY MEANS CIRCUMCISION DOESN'T WORK AS A SAFE-SEX METHOD, YOU MORONS.

Besides, let me reiterate what any sane person already knows: rolling a foreskin back in the shower is *not* rocket science. Mother Nature is smart and knows exactly what she's doing. Like an eyelid, the foreskin is a protective layer of skin the body actively needs.

In fact, it has a whopping sixteen functions, including: providing bacteriostatic action around the head, protecting the nerves to keep the penis sensitive during sex (where the foreskin also acts as a rolling device – otherwise thrusting would hurt more and feel a bit pinched), distributing natural lubricants, storing pheromones for releases on arousal – making us more attractive to our other halves on a chemical level – and acting as a sleeping bag for the shaft, keeping it safe and warm. (Intrepid explorer Ranulph Fiennes discovered this on one of his treks when it stopped him getting frostbite.)

It also has other surprising uses – it acts as a handy

grip to pull your penis out from your fly when you're in a dash at the urinals, whilst one entrepreneurial drug dealer even hid his cocaine stash in there at customs.

Maybe part of the decision to allow circumcision is psychological. We see our kids as children, never potential sexual beings, so don't bother to question how it may affect their future pleasures. This is understandable, but taking away a person's choice on something so personal as genital integrity is just asking for trouble.

The appropriately named Catherine Hood, a counsellor from the Institute of Psychosexual Medicine, sees many men who are angry about having been circumcised as a boy. She explains that they experience feelings of invasion, self-loathing and shame. 'The issues that men are angry about when they seek help are very individual,' she says from her clinic.

> Sometimes they are angry with the fact they have had the procedure and this can lead to a sense of loss or of being different to the other men they have seen. This can cause a drop in sexual confidence, avoidance of relationships, or I have seen one man who felt he had reduced sensation and so didn't enjoy sex as much as a result.

> Others are more generally angry with their parents or early life and the circumcision becomes a focus for their anger. Obviously parents make the decision to get their

children circumcised and the child doesn't have a say. If
the child then grows up with any grievance against their
parent then this is an obvious focus.

One man who grabbed the industry by the balls – and
squeezed – was William Stowell. Born and raised in New
York, he now lives in Virginia where he works, funnily
enough, as a tree surgeon. 'I climb trees with a power saw,
a rope, a saddle and a saw. I'm a third-generation cutter
on my father's side of the family,' he enthuses.

'What's funny is that girls on dates vilify me for cutting down trees. The irony of this definitely hasn't been
lost on me,' he laughs.

In 2001 he made history when he became the first man
in the world to sue his hospital of birth for removing his
foreskin without consent. 'It was something I couldn't *not*
do. I was pretty pissed off because I'd been deprived of my
natural body,' he tells me, both eloquently and without
the usual nervous energy which comes with men talking about their bodies. 'It was intuitive. I can't simplify
it any more than to say: I had a whole penis, somebody
cut part of it off, which left me with less of a penis. That's
not OK with me.'

To prove it, he fought hard and won a landmark settlement which was rumoured to have hit the $100,000
mark. At the time, he was in the military, where he served

in the Air Force, but he went on to become the poster boy for the anti-circumcision movement. His story went so viral that he ended up on *Good Morning America*, which – for the sake of us Brits – is the big time. He also appeared, fully clothed, in a couple of adult magazines like *Penthouse*, which, perhaps surprisingly, was the tipping point. At the same time, the Catholic Church started coming under fire for the molestation scandals and, being a Catholic hospital, they wanted no more drama and settled with a fat cheque.

'People always go on about the welfare of children. Oh, it's about the children, do it for the children, protect the children, they say – before slicing their son's dick open. It's a joke.' When I call the NSPCC, Save the Children and Barnado's to check this, I discover he's right – despite what we know, none of them have a single policy to protect boys from genital cutting. Even now.

'I didn't keep most of the money from my lawsuit,' William clarifies. 'I set up a trust fund to help other men sue their doctors and hospitals, because it's blatantly different treatment of genders. Girls are protected, boys are violated,' he says.

Like thousands of other men across the world, William found some relief in foreskin restoration, which involves stretching out a new fold of skin, a long process which can take years. 'It wasn't easy. Whilst growing out the skin there were times when the head wasn't always covered – and that was terribly painful,' he says.

> Sometimes the skin would roll back and just the head of my penis touching my underwear was excruciating. It felt like rubbing a wire brush against it. But it was worth it. After I started restoring myself I began to feel sensations I'd experienced when I was younger. From before my penis dried out and died in my teens.

When I ask him what these sensations are – what sex is like now with a foreskin, a foreskin which has about 20,000 compressed nerve endings, he pauses – then uses two adjectives: 'luscious' and 'juicy'. We both pause, then collapse into laughter. 'I'm fairly good with words, but there are times when words fail,' he says. 'All I know is I wouldn't go back. I don't care if some guy wants to castrate himself with a broken liquor bottle when he's eighteen, I don't give a damn – but it's about choice. He should make that decision as an adult.'

Sadly, that doesn't sit well with the other driving force behind the industry: money.

'There are at least 1 million circumcisions which take place every year in the United States: that's 3,000 per day, each of which comes at a price,' adds Jonathon Conte.

> In addition to that there are the people who make money off the tools used – the clamps, the boards used to strap down the children, the cutting utensils and the anaesthetic. On top of that there's the tissue-harvesting industry, where a number of companies make a profit on neo-natal foreskin. The tissue, after amputation, is sold to biotech companies and it's used for skin grafts, burn victims, diabetic patients, scientific research and anti-wrinkle cream.

Queen of TV, Oprah Winfrey, found herself in trouble when she endorsed a skin cream that included cells from discarded foreskins. TNS Essential Serum, made by Skin-Medica, uses foreskin fibroblast – a piece of human skin used as a culture to grow other skin or cells. She described the product, which sells for about £150 per ounce, as her 'magic fountain of youth'.

Hordes of protestors picketed her outside TV studios nationwide, some with eloquent placards which read: 'Circumcise Oprah! She'll be "cleaner"'. Couldn't have said it better myself.

'It's a huge multi-million-dollar industry, so there's a lot of financial incentive to keep the circumcision train rolling,' adds Conte. 'There are many people who are making a lot of money when it happens, who would make no money if it didn't. Forget human rights, it's all about the mighty dollar.'

Which begs the question: is there a hidden financial reason why we're encouraged to cut our sons? Is this just a cash-generator – straight from his pants? Are we lining the pockets of fat cats who treat our lads like a commodity? In short, yes. Which makes the whole process even more sinister. Not least because parents are supposed to protect their offspring, not serve them up on a platter.

When I broach this with William, he admits that – beyond everything – what his circumcision ultimately hurt was his relationship with his mother, who allowed it to happen.

> I'm a father now, I have a daughter, but I still feel to this day that my mother could've done a much better job of protecting me. What she did was unforgivable. I'm not one of these people who can easily forgive and forget, but especially not about something like that.

In therapist-speak, this is probably referred to as the breakthrough. Because here William gets to the heart of the matter, offering perhaps the best ever reason not to circumcise your child.

Otherwise, not only are you letting Tony the Tiger's creator affect his future sex life, which is just weird, but you're also cutting more than human flesh. You're potentially severing the priceless bond with your perfect son.

Nothing is worth that.

EVERYDAY BULLSHIT

THERE'S A CONSTANT NARRATIVE ABOUT men in the modern world, mostly critical – and curated by everyone except us.

Fortunately, as we're the ultimate authority on ourselves, it's us – nobody else – who gets to have the final say on matters of masculinity.

So, as we're long overdue a reality check, let's do some conscious uncoupling from the everyday bullshit of being a bloke.

CHIVALRY

In short, don't buy it. No, seriously – don't pick up that tab! At a time when young women are solvent, self-sufficient and frequently out-earning their male counterparts (the Chartered Management Institute found that female managers in their twenties are now earning 2.1 per cent more than men of the same age) we should help them enjoy the fruits of their labour. Especially on dates, where the boundaries of a relationship are defined early.

This doesn't have to be a romance-free divide of who had the biggest starter, but a mutually kind sharing of plates – as well as minds – is just plain polite.

Typically, social etiquette dictates that the 'asker' funds the first date, whilst the 'ask-ee' gets the second, so feel free to follow this blueprint – but do it in a coffee shop where everything's a bit more low-key. Stop the naff, overstated gestures of Michelin-starred restaurants for a first date. You're not Donald Trump and you don't even know if she's even worth it yet. She might order three courses and a bottle of wine and then sit there – lobotomised – when the bill arrives.

Instead, take her for a caffeine hit somewhere original and be generous there. The gesture is the same, as is the level of respect for another person's time, but the financial impact is not. It also suggests casual parity and looks a lot less desperate than booking the best table somewhere like the Chiltern Firehouse, which, BTW, is totally over now Bono's been.

From here you're free to upgrade accordingly because, by this point, you'll know you're paying for somebody who treats you (and your wallet) with a bit of decorum. After all, if she's not a sex object, you're not a success object. Everybody wins.

Naturally, plenty of women already go dutch. Plenty more settle the tab altogether. We like these women. A lot. We like them more when they allow us to treat them – and, likewise, when they spoil us. I just wish they'd be less discreet and a bit more consistent, because over the months it took me to write this book I observed hundreds of men financing dinners in fancy places, whilst their glamorous guests froze at the presentation of the credit card machine – even though, decorated with expensive handbags and bodies contorted into various post-surgical poses, they could clearly afford to cough up.

Besides, it wasn't so long ago that opening doors,

offering seats and paying for dates was branded 'benev-olent sexism' – which is seriously scraping the bottom of the hardship barrel. Personally, it made me think of Bart Simpson's sage advice when he noted 'you're damned if you do and you're damned if you don't'.

So, quite simply, ditch the chivalry act and save such welcome efforts for your friends. You are *not* desperate.

That said, there are certainly some undercurrents of chivalry that are worth keeping. These are otherwise referred to as: 'being nice'. Holding a door open just makes the minutiae of daily life a bit easier for everyone (apart from that awkward moment when there are loads in a row and you run out of ways to say thank you). Even Hulk Hogan, who could probably rip the thing off its hinges, would be grateful for somebody extending such basic courtesy, because it's not really about whether he could muster the strength to hold it open. It's just being decent.

If anything, the bigger issue is age, not sex. In parts of Asia, pensioners are revered. Here, they're allowed to soil themselves whilst a 'carer' nicks £20 from their purse. So here's an idea: chivalry ultimately means putting the other person first, even just for a second. So, as we can all do this regardless of our hormone group, let's start by being nice to our elders and our youngsters first, then work our way inwards.

This way, everybody wins in order. Men and women together.

WORKING DADS

It's a mathematical fact there aren't enough hours in the day for anyone, male or female, to work sixty-hour weeks, all year, raise children and run a house full-time. So the idea that it should be split down the middle to prove some political point might sound right-on, but – in reality – it's the cause of so much unnecessary marital conflict.

Instead, let's be realistic. Whether it's an unwelcome truth or not, most new mothers like to nurture the baby they've been carrying for nine months, whilst fathers typically return to work and help bankroll it.

THIS IS ABSOLUTELY OK.

Think about it: women carry life. That's the ultimate. We can't compete with that, so our purpose is to provide *for* that life. That's our identity as fathers and what we bring to the table. It's been this way since time immemorial because it's cost-effective, practical and sensible. Recent legislative changes tried to rewrite this fact when the coalition brought in extended paternity leave in 2011, taking it beyond the standard two weeks, but it failed miserably. Fewer than one in fifty used it. In fact, for various reasons, a quarter of new fathers took no leave at all.

THIS IS ALSO ABSOLUTELY OK IF IT'S WHAT EACH HOUSEHOLD WANTS.

Eventually, in every relationship, somebody will need to take the bulk of one responsibility, whilst the other manages the rest. Personally, I don't care who assumes the traditional breadwinner role, but unless you can afford a nanny (or manny) to do it for you, you'll need to face the prickly modern dilemma of parental roles.

Whatever the outcome, just remember: it's a toss-up between you and your partner, *not* a coin-flip adjudicated by topless banshees from FEMEN. I say this because whenever working fathers are discussed in the media, the insinuation is that they don't pull their weight.

Actually, the opposite is true: aside from proving we can multi-task just fine, research collated by the Fatherhood Institute shows British dads work the longest hours in Europe – an average of 46.9 hours per week, compared with 45.5 hours in Portugal, 41.5 hours in Germany and 40 hours in France. Around one in eight UK fathers work excessively long hours – 60 or more – whilst almost 40 per cent graft more than 48 hours each week, so – contrary to popular opinion – we don't leave the house every morning to ride the Venga Bus and shag our secretaries.

In fact, we're spending more time with our children than ever.

In the late 1990s, dads of children under five were devoting an average of two hours per day on child-related activities, compared to less than fifteen minutes in the mid-1970s.

Today, fathers' time spent with their children currently accounts for one-third of total parental childcare, so there.

THE PATRIARCHY™

For decades therapists have listened to people blame their parents for their own mentalisms – because it's easier to abdicate personal responsibility and blame a more powerful presence.

On a much bigger, more pernicious scale, that's exactly what modern society does with men and theories of The Patriarchy™. But, hang on, does it even exist?

'We have never really lived in a "patriarchy" the way feminists have historically defined it,' says *VICE* magazine-featured activist Karen Straughan.

> Whilst feminists will point to CEOs, politicians and people in positions of enormous power and

responsibility, they don't so much acknowledge the power of lobby groups to sway those politicians. When it comes to gender issues, women have the more powerful lobby. Just look at abortion, birth control, divorce law and custody issues etc. The men's lobby is virtually non-existent. In fact, in many cases, men depend on the campaigning of women, like myself.

In other words, even if we do live in a patriarchy, it's a gynocentric one that prioritises the care of women. After all, they may have fought for the vote, but men still have it taken away if they don't sign up for military draft.

If ordinary men only have their problems addressed when women speak up for them, and when politicians can be convinced those problems also harm mothers and children, then the 'patriarchy' feminists envision does not exist. It is not a system that benefits men at the expense of women.

There may have been a patriarchy at some point in history, but it has never been a system that oppresses women for men's express benefit. And whatever form of patriarchy might have existed, it's now almost entirely eradicated in the West.

THE SENTENCING GAP

Just when you think you've heard the last truly absurd idea, another appears right before you – like the cognitive equivalent of a corrupt MP (or his equally corrupt wife).

Believe it or not, the latest brain fail is the campaign for all women's prisons to be closed. Yep, you read that correctly. In 2007, Frances Crook, the director of the Howard League for Penal Reform, was quoted in *The Guardian* as saying: 'For women who offend, prison simply doesn't work. It is time to end the use of traditional prisons for women.'

Since then, the debate has continually rambled on – which is impressive considering it doesn't actually have any merit and we're all supposed to be equal.

Apparently, in her eyes, jailing violent offenders – you know, murderers, paedophiles and arsonists – is utterly counterproductive if they have a penchant for Meg Ryan films. Instead, female felons should be free-range, purely because they're women. WHICH ISN'T REMOTELY SEXIST OR GENDER PROFILING, of course.

Personally, this theory alone might be worthy of a custodial sentence, not least because we already know it doesn't work.

In the early 1970s London's Holloway Prison was completely demolished and rebuilt after hardcore feminists asserted that women only commit crimes because of a) men and b) momentary mental illness – which could be cured with lots of hand-holding and group therapy.

So, at an estimated cost of £6 million, a new hospital-like prison was opened in 1977 to lead the future of correctional reform for female offenders. Except it was all bollocks and – forty years on – there are more Holloway inmates than ever and the building is a dump. Awkward.

Yes, it's very unfortunate that people end up in jail, but they're generally in there for a reason. Besides, these institutions make our lives better by keeping scary people off the streets, including – at one point – Martha Stewart, which further proves my point. Have you seen the American version of *The Apprentice*? She's terrifying.

Besides, without women's prisons we wouldn't have *Orange Is the New Black* or the criminally underrated *Brokedown Palace* – which would be a shame. OK, maybe I'm not selling this, but what I am saying is: prisons are democratic. Nobody is above the law. Not by class, race or sex. That's the whole point.

More pertinently, what exactly are these campaigners worrying about? Few women are jailed anyway – unlike men. Last October, during a House of Commons debate on the topic of female sentencing, MP Philip Davies delivered a rapid-fire critique of the way UK courts frequently go easy on women.

A transcript of the debate, which can be found online at parliament.uk, is fourteen pages long and lines up false assumptions like beer cans on a fence, which he shoots down – bang! – with fact.

Specifically, he found that more men were sentenced to immediate custody in every offence group, in every court, in every part of the country – for *exactly* the same crimes. The figures, compiled and verified by the Home Office, show that 34.7 per cent of male offenders were sentenced to immediate custody for offences involving violence against a person compared to only 16.9 per cent of women.

Similarly 44.9 per cent of men went straight to prison for committing a burglary compared to 26.6 per cent of women, as well as 61.7 per cent of male robbers compared to just 37.7 per cent of female robbers.

One of the excuses for this is that women are so controlled by men they only break the law because we tell them to – a bit like ASBO Stepford Wives. Not only is this seriously undermining a woman's brain power and autonomy, but – if it were true – we'd also be saying that men are responsible for all the terrible things in the world, which can't be true when you consider the Falklands War, *Loose Women* and Mumsnet.

All equally devastating, all led by women. Enough said.

THE JAY-Z EFFECT

Who knows what happened in that lift? No, seriously, who knows? I want the details. Now.

Not just to satisfy my morbid curiosity, but so I can write a huge take-down piece on Solange Knowles, who clearly still hasn't understood what she did wrong.

It's perhaps ironic that Beyoncé's little sister can't score a hit in the charts, but can on her brother-in-law – then again, he was an easy target, being both male and in an enclosed space. Fortunately, if her music career does continue to flounder, at least she has a future in comedy, because, apparently, the whole incident was H-I-L-A-R-I-O-U-S!

Camilla Long, journalist at *The Times*, wrote on Twitter: 'HA HA HA. I love the way he grabs her foot, as if that's somehow going to power things down.' Meanwhile, Caitlin Moran added: 'I AM OBSESSED WITH THIS VIDEO … Her shoe comes off in his groin. She's going for it.'

I check myself over and – no, sorry – still not laughing.

Perhaps *The Observer*'s Barbara Ellen will show me the light. She's always fun. 'It's important to note that what happened in the lift was *not* domestic violence,' she asserts unconvincingly. Not least because a) that's exactly how she defined Charles Saatchi grabbing Nigella Lawson's neck and b) the Home Office themselves describe it as: 'Any incident or threatening behaviour, violence or abuse (psychological, physical, sexual, financial or emotional) between adults who are or have been intimate partners or are family members, regardless of gender or sexuality.'

Oh. But I have faith. With a Jerry Maguire-type voice in my head I think, 'Come on Barbara. Show. Me. The. FUNNY!' and read on. 'Some females might have periods in their life when they get "slap-happy", primarily when socialising, maybe when attention-seeking, usually when drunk (guilty!),' she continues.

No, still not laughing. Instead, my instinct is to close all the windows in my house and scream very loudly into a cushion that Barbara Ellen is the c-word, but I refrain: purely because I doubt she has the depth or the warmth.

What I do decide would be more productive is to detail precisely why there's no punchline – ever – in men being their partner's punchbag. Especially when up-to-date, verified numbers from the Office for National Statistics, courtesy of charity Mankind, show that:

- 38 per cent of domestic abuse victims are male: for every five victims, three will be women, two will be men.

- More married men suffered from partner abuse in 2012/13 than married women.

- Of those, more men suffered from severe force than women.

- 21 per cent of men and 21 per cent of women suffered three or more incidents of partner abuse in 2012/13.

To be fair, it's not just Caitlin, Camilla and Babs who promulgate this attitude: it's endemic. When footage of the infamous Met Ball assault leaked, the internet was flooded with memes making light of the matter, each compiled on major news sites around the world as light entertainment, when actually it was just offensive. Especially when we consider that it's long been known that men are almost equal victims of domestic violence and any difference in physical strength between men and women can easily be neutralised with either a weapon or the element of surprise.

Maybe Erin Pizzey was correct when, during an interview in her London home about the academic and industry-wide deceit that has long gone on around domestic violence, she told me: 'This is a huge, million-pound industry and those women who control it are not willing to share it.'

Then again, maybe I'm reading too much into it. Perhaps I'm just suffering a severe sense-of-humour failure and need to lighten up. You know, see the funny side. To check this, I watch the infamous, grainy footage online and concur that, yep – sorry gentlemen – the girls were right about this one. It turns out the entire incident was a laugh-out-loud scream.

Just like when Chris Brown hit Rihanna, right?

'MAN FLU'

Along with 'man up' or 'grow a pair', the term 'man flu' is officially our enemy in a cold war.

Sure, it's just a lark which happened to raise one forced chuckle, once, ten years ago, but now it's becoming a standard seasonal misery.

Firstly, it's not funny. Secondly, and more importantly, people who use it aren't laughing *with* us – they're laughing *at* us. It's the snide suggestion that men are big babies for feeling the physical effects of a virus which might make carrying 200lb of muscle and fat a bit trickier. And, according to experts, it does.

Neuroscientists have proved we suffer more acute forms of cold and flu than women because of our preoptic nucleus and extra temperature receptors in the brain, or something.

Besides, it's not man flu. It's not even real influenza. What you have is a cold.

THE TERM 'INDEPENDENT WOMAN'

Seriously, I respect anyone who works hard and is solvent, but what do these people expect – a medal? For being self-sufficient? THEY'RE SUPPOSED TO BE INDEPENDENT. FOREVER.

It's called adulthood.

BEING 'A REAL MAN'

Are you a fictional character? No. Are you a male human being aged eighteen or over? Yes. Congratulations, you're a real man.

BEING MALE OR FEMALE IS A SOCIAL CONSTRUCT

No, it isn't. It's an evolved biological trait called sexual dimorphism, resulting from mate selection – which is the sole reason we're all here. This means that sex isn't a social construct, but rather society is built – and developed – on the combined, complementary differences between the sexes.

WAR

Never a cheery subject, war gets even grimmer when you realise it almost completely skipped the equality drive.

Hillary Clinton once said – remarkably, with a straight face – that women have 'always been the primary victims of war', not the men who get their legs blown off on the battlefield in Iraq. Or Libya. Or Sudan.

'Women lose their husbands, their fathers, their sons in combat,' she continued. 'Women often have to flee from the only homes they have ever known. Women are often left with the responsibility, alone, of raising the children.'

Er, with all due respect, Hillary, this does not a primary victim maketh.

Indeed, she has a point that everybody is affected by conflict in one way or another, but let's keep it real here: it's men who bear the brunt of warfare, both in action and in administration.

Despite the slew of equality legislation which has passed in recent years, American men are still forced – by law – to register for military conscription or face punishment, whilst women are not. Here in Britain the debate on whether females should serve on the front line also persists, even though I'm not sure what there is to discuss. We know women are equal to men and that a grenade is going to hurt no matter who throws it.

One argument that's regularly presented is that women shouldn't serve because they might have children – or, at some point in the future, go on to have children. I sympathise. But, then again, I tend to think anyone dying for somebody else's war is unfortunate, especially parents, so surely the solution is simply to draft both men and women on the condition they're childless. Currently, Norway is the only European country to agree this is fair.

This aside, men frankly deserve a break. We've been at it since about 3000 BC and it's still going on. OK, a lot of it was started by men, but only to protect the rest of the world from a greater threat. Veterans didn't sign up because the trenches looked like those log cabins in Centre Parcs. They had no choice. Plus, women used to give young lads a white feather as a symbol of cowardice if they hadn't 'done their duty' and been shipped off. Think slut-shaming, but in reverse – and with death as the alternative.

That said, we don't help ourselves. Men everywhere still have this weird instinct to be chivalrous about war. Our steeped-in-instinct hearts haven't caught up with our modernised brains. When singer Bryan Adams diverted from pop into photography and made a coffee-table book called *Wounded: The Legacy of War*, he held a launch at the National Portrait Gallery in Trafalgar Square. Featuring a number of disabled soldiers, it definitely wasn't bedtime reading – in fact, it was in-your-face, distressing, naked combat reality. Some of the featured soldiers had legs missing, others arms blown off. One was blinded when shrapnel from an explosion ripped through his eyelids, whilst another suffered head-to-toe burns so severe he was left unrecognisable to friends and family.

All of them were present at the party, which it made it very emotionally charged. At one point I had to leave the room when I thanked a veteran – Sergeant Rick Clement, 1st Battalion Duke of Lancaster's Regiment – for his service. He was just thirty years old when he lost both legs in Afghanistan, where he was on a two-pronged mission: first, to disrupt the Taliban from their training and, secondly, to help local communities with teaching and education.

'It was a normal morning and we were going out on patrol,' he recounts in the book.

> We pushed out as standard ... the guy with the metal detector was out front, another guy was covering him and I always liked to lead near to them, but the Taliban had started using no-metal-content IEDs, which weren't picked up.
>
> I was conscious during the explosion, but don't really remember seeing anything. My legs had gone. They were both blown clean off. My right leg is a high-above-knee

amputation; I've got a stump left. My left leg was taken all the way up to my hip, so there's nothing there. I had a lot of internal injuries, too. My genitals were badly burned, kind of into the right side of my leg, but I've had an operation to reverse all that. My bodily functions were also affected, both urinating and defecating … but, still, I owe it to the guys who didn't make it home to make the most of what I've got.

His story is gut-wrenching. Just like all the other men featured in the book. And, with the exception of one brave woman, it's exactly that: all men. Just like the Great War which saw TEN MILLION MEN die (yet the recent BBC coverage of the 100-year anniversary devoted countless time to 'women's contribution'). However, when I ask Bryan what he thought of it all – the loss, the bravery, the ratio of men to women and whether this would ever change – he didn't have the balls to admit that, even in terms of the injured and fallen, war is primarily a major, ballistic men's issue.

It's. A. Fact.

Yes, ideally there would be no war, and, yes, there are women who suffer and contribute invaluably, and, yes, it's mainly men with bad ideas who start wars in the first place – but the main victims have historically been – and largely remain – young, innocent lads.

The same guys who are the worst-performing demographic in UK schools. Half of these lads, who are constantly told they're privileged despite not actually having anything, aren't turning down managerial jobs at Barclays in favour of signing up. They're choosing it because their only other option is a 'career' with a tabard in a supermarket.

And, let's be honest, how many men get laid saying they work in ASDA?

THE VOTE

People love rewriting history when it comes to the vote because it paints a convenient picture of bad male establishment versus good female underclass, which requires no effort to comprehend.

Sadly, it's a distortion of truth – which is why it needs correcting here. Trigger warning: the following contains fact.

Believing they were appointed by God, kings and queens once ruled the land single-handedly. However, because one man (or woman) cannot rule alone, a royal council of elite advisors (all landed gentry) was set up to assist them. King John started this in 1215 with Magna Carta and it gradually became Parliament, but back then it was heavily restricted. For example, they could only meet when he said so, rendering them the political equivalent of backing singers.

Only the very rich owned property then, so this became the voting prerequisite. It was an easy way to maintain the status quo and ensure that big, important decisions were made by aristocratic landowners with similar interests, not the local plebs.

People were working their fingers to the bone and generating lots of wealth for the country, but getting little political acknowledgement in return.

To avoid the threat of civil unrest, the state ushered in the 1832 Representation of the People Act, but – still – only a tiny minority of men could vote.

However, central Parliament was largely niche back then – people didn't pay taxes to it because there was no welfare state or government-funded education system. So, instead, local councils managed these matters regionally. Brilliantly, many women frequently voted in parish elections and held local office during the Victorian era.

That said, big, national decisions were still only made by the elite. The revolution happened with the arrival of the First World War in 1914, which changed everything. At the time, the average woman wouldn't vote in central government, but nor could the average man – yet it was men (and only men – of all classes) who were drafted into battle.

Incredibly, roughly half of the six million men who fought in the First World War could not vote. Why? Because the biggest factor in voting eligibility was class, not gender.

When the horrors of the war were finally over, the government owed us big time, so – in 1918, the same year the First World War ended – the law was relaxed to give all men over twenty-one and all women over thirty the vote, although the latter was dependent on being a member of the Local Government Register (or married to somebody who was), a property owner or a graduate voting in a university constituency.

But, given that young men – and only young men – fought on the front line, this was fair.

'On an historical timescale, the enfranchisement of men hardly preceded that of women significantly,' says writer William Collins, who edits a site clarifying the reality behind gender politics.

Much is made in some quarters that the 1918 Act did not give the vote to women at age twenty-one. But the reason is clear. Women outnumbered men before the war, and outnumbered them even more emphatically afterwards by virtue of the war deaths. It was thought inappropriate to introduce women immediately as the majority voters, especially in view of the hardships men had faced in the trenches. Only ten years later, women became the majority of voters and remain so to this day.

Likewise, Parliament was all-male when the 1918 amendment was made, so the idea that women's suffrage was forced from the male grip is false – they enthusiastically passed it by 385 votes in favour to fifty-five against.

Introducing the reform, then Home Secretary George Cave said:

> War by all classes of our countrymen has brought us nearer together, has opened men's eyes, and removed misunderstandings on all sides. It has made it, I think, impossible that ever again, at all events in the lifetime of the present generation, there should be a revival of the old class feeling which was responsible for so much, and, among other things, for the exclusion for a period, of so many of our population from the class of electors. I think I need say no more to justify this extension of the franchise.

It was a game-changer. And within ten years all men and all women could vote at twenty-one, which means that both sexes got it at (roughly) the same time.

'The true history of women's suffrage is the working-class struggle,' adds Collins.

> Universal suffrage came about due to the breakdown of the old electoral system after WWI. There was unanimous agreement that the men at war must have the vote on their return. The only credible option was to adopt enfranchisement as a right for all men over a certain age. The motivation was genuinely egalitarian, a spirit engendered by the war.
>
> Once votes for all men was an agreed principle, votes for women followed virtually as an automatic consequence – because the disenfranchisement of working-class men had been the political barrier to the enfranchisement of women. Hence, that women got the vote owes more to the Kaiser than to the Pankhursts.

The great irony, he adds, is that women could've achieved the vote much earlier if they'd actually campaigned for both sexes to be fully emancipated, rather than just themselves (which you could say they still do to this day).

'The suffragettes' gender-specific perspective was only because they did not recognise the equal rights of working-class men, who were also largely disenfranchised,' he says.

> This is one of those horrible twists of fate by which we

> are taunted. Present-day feminists are culpable because
> – even with the leisure to put the history into proper
> focus – they still insist on regarding the suffragettes as
> triumphing over the hegemony of men. The orthodox
> feminist narrative is not only inaccurate but disguises a
> horrible, if unintentional, truth: that the vote for women
> resulted from the wholesale slaughter of men.

Granted, this might sound gauche – but it's true. The very least we can do is respect their sacrifice by remembering it accurately.

WAGE GAP

For years, men have been guilt-tripped over a gender pay gap that apparently sees women lose thousands of pounds in a salary disparity.

The great news? According to experts who actually understand it, it simply isn't true.

I know, I know – that's tricky to comprehend. A bit like when somebody first tells you about infinity. But stick with it because the claim has been debunked by some of the most world-renowned economists, including Claudia Goldin and Lawrence Katz, both Economics

Professors at Harvard University, not to mention boy-bashing Hanna Roisin (!) who all similarly rejected it on the basis that its calculation is socially and mathematically flawed.

'The wage gap myth has been repeatedly discredited but it will not die,' says Christina Hoff-Somers, resident scholar at the American Enterprise Institute and presenter of YouTube's 'The Factual Feminist'. 'The 23 per cent gap is the difference between *average* earnings for *all* men and *all* women, but it does NOT take into account differences in occupation, expertise, job tenure and hours worked. When it does, the so-called wage gap narrows to the point of vanishing.'

Essentially, this means a woman who works as a primary school teacher isn't going to be paid the same as a man who works as a brain surgeon. WHICH IS HOW IT SHOULD BE. This gap isn't about black-and-white institutional bias based on gender, but category, profession and salaries structured on skill, difficulty and reward.

It also means that you've been lied to for decades.

> It's all down to life decisions. Young men at university tend to graduate in the top ten most lucrative subjects, whereas women populate the least profitable – social work or primary school teaching. All

the evidence suggests that, although women have the talents for engineering and computer science, their interests tend to lie elsewhere. To say these women are helplessly enthralled into sexist stereotypes or manipulated into their life choices is divorced from reality – and insulting. If a woman wants to be a teacher, more power to her.

That's not to say there still isn't anecdotal evidence of it, of course – there are certainly some existing cases – but, ultimately, the issue isn't real, so please stop believing it so faithfully. Many women work fewer hours than men. Many choose comfortable, low-paying jobs rather than strenuous, dangerous and life-threatening ones. These naturally bring higher pay for men, but – according to the Office for National Institute of Occupational Safety and Health – also put male workplace fatalities at 94 per cent of the total.

Besides, it's not always to the disadvantage of women. Ever seen Wimbledon? Men and women historically got paid different prize sums because they ultimately played for different periods of time: women less, men more. Now, women get exactly the same prize money as men – but aren't asked to do the same work, which technically means they earn more per hour.

'I've long argued from looking at UK pay figures that

what we have is not a gender-based pay gap at all, but a motherhood one,' says financial expert Tim Worstall.

> Lesbians on average earn more than men, as do never-married childless women, but what 'gap' there is opens up around the age of thirty, which is also the average age of primagravidae – a woman's first pregnancy. It was exactly my analysis of the problem that led to the introduction of shared parental leave in the UK. I can even introduce you to the political activist I convinced and the process by which it went from an idea to being on the law books.

Either way, it's women – not men – who get to spend the majority of money that's earned by households, which means consumption inequality runs entirely in women's favour, so the issue is dead and gone.

In other words, with the exception of some real-but-rare cases on both sides, the pay gap is just spin, which is why it's important to remember exactly where these messages originate from. Do they stem from an independent financial body – or a women's society that needs to keep feminism relevant to justify their existence?

'The basic proof it's not all due to some evil patriarchy is that if businesses actually could pay women 77 cents on the dollar for the same work, they'd just hire women. There would be no reason to ever hire men, but that clearly isn't what's happening,' says Isaac Cohen, *Forbes* journalist. 'Businesses really, really want women. It's great PR.'

VIDEO GAMES

Yep, according to the gender police, 'Gamergate' is the latest grievance against us, with claims the industry is inherently biased and fosters sexism.

This is despite the fact many computer games are made, and consumed, by women. So what's the reality?

'Modern feminists claim women are pigeon-holed into clichés which objectify them, but this an entirely negative, subjective interpretation,' says online gaming guru George 'Maddox' Ouzounian.

> These people have a laser-focus on whether women are treated like decoration or sexual objects in video games, but they ignore how men are maimed and slaughtered. In classic side-scrolling action games of the late '80s, for example, such as Contra and Commando, the player kills male soldiers almost exclusively. Men are stabbed, shot with machine guns, lasers, flame throwers, grenades etc. at such an astonishing rate, it quite literally makes them expendable.

In Super Mario Bros none of the characters have any free agency, least of all Mario, who's literally being controlled by players all around the world – both male and female. Mario has no free will and you can kill him over and over again if you want to. Does that dehumanise Mario? And what does it even mean to humanise a fictional object like Mario? Does it matter? Does it have a real-world impact? If so, how large of a contribution to this impact do these games have? And what evidence is there for this impact? These questions aren't explored by feminists, which makes their criticism hollow at best, and disingenuous at worst.

Agreed. So, if male characters also get a rough ride, why are objectors causing such a stink?

'It seems to be about relevance,' he adds.

First- and second-wave feminism was so successful that it largely rendered the modern movement and its acolytes irrelevant.

Professors, authors and social critics feel the need to surface so-called 'hidden' sexism in the media we consume to make a case for their existence. Many people have made a good living from gender theory, and they may feel that their jobs are threatened.

The modern feminism movement is an amalgam of

all three, but frustratingly, there is no consensus among them over what women should or shouldn't do, how they should or shouldn't be represented, and whether or not a perceived threat is indeed bad for women or just that: a perception held by a minority of women.

MICRO-AGGRESSIONS

This is one of the many wacky, esoteric terms to have gone mainstream. It claims to define non-verbal, unintentional 'slights' against anyone – and I mean anyone – who isn't a white man.

But, hang on, if these alleged insults are truly micro, then surely the corresponding 'trauma' is equally minuscule – and thus not worth discussing?

Exactly.

DOUBLE STANDARDS

Oh, where to begin on this one!

First up, quotas. Vince Cable may have recently declared them tantamount to sexual discrimination

– and he's right – but, actually, I quite like the idea. Then again, I also think they should be applied consistently and equally across the board. Not just in boardrooms where you get nice pay-offs and lots of power, but also on battlefields and oil rigs, coal mines and abattoirs. After all, people bemoan the number of men getting to the top of their game, but conveniently ignore the overwhelming number at the bottom, too.

Given that schools are failing boys but most of them are female-dominated, quotas for male teachers should also probably be introduced here. After all, most men won't go near a primary classroom because they're petrified of being branded sex pests. A little bit of formal encouragement would combat this rather nicely.

Outside the workplace, one-rule-for-all should still apply. Even if just online.

When the Women Who Eat on Tubes group sparked controversy for trending with 21,000 members last year, humourless haters claimed it encouraged people to 'objectify and humiliate women' who were unaware of their image being taken whilst masticating in public.

Typically, men were painted as perverts for laughing at a woman forcing down a fajita, yet the professionally offended ignored the fact that half of them were women – taking photos, uploading pictures, commenting. They also forget about the existence of TubeCrush: a website which, for years, has encouraged women to upload pictures of attractive men using the London Underground and communally gush over them online.

When it launched in 2011 it was lauded as a peaktime pastime by everything from Pinterest to the *Evening Standard*, who wrote a fawning feature about it, saying:

> Flirty females are using their smartphones to capture the dishiest of the Underground's two million daily commuters, and uploading the unsuspecting men onto hit website TubeCrush.net. The cute commuters are then rated and commented on by admiring women – with surveys taken as to which Tube lines have the hottest men (so far, overwhelmingly, the Northern line is winning).

Disturbingly, some of the lads in the photographs didn't always look old enough to be sixteen, whilst others – wearing shorts in the summer – were snapped sitting down as the material rode up their legs. Creepy, right?

Brilliantly, the solution is always simple: laugh, hysterically – then join in.

I was once travelling on the Northern line when a young woman was trying to surreptitiously take a photograph of a man in a suit. Hilariously, her flash went off – at which point he started photographing her, saying he was going to put the pictures online – which caused her to scurry off at the next stop in shame and frustration.

That's because what he did is exactly what the Women Eating blog does – it holds a mirror up to all the double standards, and levels the playing field. Which, after all, is surely what everyone wants. Especially with revenge porn, which – if applied fairly – will surely see the women who sold naked pictures of Leicester City striker David Nugent or *Made in Chelsea*'s Spencer Matthews to the press jailed and given a criminal record.

After all, fair's fair.

BECOMING OBSOLETE

Now for the *really* good news: we aren't facing extinction.

For decades there's been fear-mongering that our fundamental Y gene is weakening to the point of redundancy, which will eventually see men become extinct. Both scientists and cultural commentators, including Michael Moore in *Stupid White Men*, have been fantasising over the idea, predicting the collapse of men over an embarrassing five-million year descent into nullity.

Fortunately, it turns out – rather nicely – that it's a complete myth.

A recent study conducted by boffins at UCL, Oxford University and the Swedish Agricultural University, published in the *Proceedings of the National Academy of Sciences* journal, found that we aren't genetic wastelands after all. Instead, we're here to stay.

Sorry, ladies, you'd better cancel that party bus.

A similar project in the USA, which looked at the genetics of rhesus macaque monkeys, found that whilst male DNA did shed some characteristics some time ago, it has since stabilised. Which means our clever Y chromosome simply decluttered.

Biology professor David Page, of the Whitehead Institute for Biomedical Research in Cambridge, Massachusetts, said:

> For the past ten years the one dominant storyline in public discourse about the Y is that it's disappearing. Putting aside the question of whether this ever had a sound scientific basis in the first place, it was a story that went viral – fast. And stayed viral.
>
> Yes, the Y was in freefall early on and genes were lost at an incredibly rapid rate. But then it levelled off – and it's been doing just fine since.

His lab researcher, Jennifer Hughes, who previously found proof that the human Y chromosome has been stable for at least 6 million years, added: 'We've been carefully developing this clear-cut way of demystifying the evolution of the Y chromosome. Now our empirical data flies in the face of all the other theories out there. I challenge anyone to argue with it.'

Time to get the drinks in, then.

THE IMPORTANCE
OF BEING EARNEST
(ABOUT ANONYMITY)

WHEN GILLIAN FLYNN'S *GONE GIRL* became a literary sensation – and, later, a global cinematic success – the illiberal left were furious that [spoiler alert!] its lead protagonist, Amy Dunne, was a woman who avenged her husband's infidelity by framing him for murder, stealing his sperm and lying about rape. Such characterisation, it seemed, deviated from the pre-approved script on what we're allowed to think, say and feel – even about fictional people who happen to be female.

Television producer David Cox claimed it 'revamps gender stereotypes – for the worse', *The Guardian*'s Emine Saner questioned whether it was 'misogynist agit-prop' and one blogger decried it as 'the crystallisation of a thousand misogynist myths and fears about female behaviour'. Not to be outdone, Vulture said 'Yes, *Gone Girl* has a woman problem', whilst Joan Smith waded into the fray, accusing the film of being a 'disgusting distortion' of truth whilst 'recycling the most egregious myths about gender-based violence' – specifically, that 'it's childishly easy to get away with making false [rape] allegations'.

Except, whilst they're all entitled to their opinions, me thinks they doth protest too much – although it's only art, it's art that imitates life for countless men across the world. Thus, if there's one area of modern manhood that demands a serious chapter in this book – above health, fatherhood, suicide and circumcision, all of which remain fiercely front-line – it's the human right to be innocent until proven guilty in a court of law.

Currently, under British legislation, any man – me, you, your father, son, brother or best friend – can be accused of rape and named by every media platform in the country, even before police bring charges. This might be acceptable if every allegation was legitimate, but, sadly, they are not. Hence, due process – and, in particular, pre-conviction anonymity – is crucial for preserving the credibility and humanity of justice.

This is particularly true when legal professionals themselves make false claims…

In June 2014, trainee barrister Rhiannon Brooker was jailed for three years after falsely accusing her former boyfriend Paul Fensome of rape and assault. He was held in custody for thirty-six days, including time on a secure wing after rumours circulated that he was a paedophile. He has since received £38,000 in compensation for the trauma.

In April 2012, Kent's Kirsty Sowden, a former John Lewis shop assistant, was jailed for crying rape over a fully consensual encounter with a man she'd met online after advertising herself as a 'BSDM princess'. He was arrested at his workplace in front of colleagues and detained in a cell, wasting 376 hours of police time to the tune of £14,000. The reason? She felt guilty for cheating on her long-term boyfriend.

Shortly after this, twenty-year-old Hannah Byron was spared jail after falsely accusing her ex-boyfriend of rape in revenge for breaking up with her. Then, Sheffield's Emma Saxon was given a custodial sentence for her second spurious claim against partner Martin Blood. He was held in police custody for fourteen hours and subjected to an intrusive medical examination – all because he'd stood her up.

Capping them all, Southampton's Elizabeth Jones was finally jailed in February – but only after making her *eleventh* false allegation. Take note, Joan Smith.

Despite these countless cases – which, admittedly, aren't the typical experience – there's a steadfast belief that men deserve the stain of rape stigma, guilty or not, simply because they are male. Writer Julie Bindel once said that 'a fair number of celebrities … have been accused of rape in the past and do not seem to have suffered longer-term. To say that an accusation ruins lives is perhaps a sweeping generalisation.' (Then again, she also wrote a sister article in *The Guardian* entitled 'Why I Hate Men', so perhaps her judgement isn't totally credible.)

Likewise, writing in the *New Statesman*, Willard Foxton denounced mutual anonymity because 'the fashionable thing to do on being cleared of rape these days is to walk free from the courtroom or police station and loudly issue a public statement calling for those accused of rape to be granted anonymity by the courts because of your "ordeal"'.

Perhaps these people should speak to Reg Traviss, the former boyfriend of Amy Winehouse, who suffered a malicious, fictitious claim in December 2012. Thankfully, he was acquitted, but only after his character had been publicly assassinated by the press, who sneered 'there's no smoke without fire'. During the case, London's Southwark Crown Court heard that his accuser was 'so drunk she couldn't stand up or walk' which many assumed to be true – until CCTV footage secured by Traviss's brother (*not* the police) proved otherwise.

Then there's Peter Bacon. In 2009, a jury cleared him of rape in just forty-five minutes after being falsely accused by a one-night stand. Yet, despite being exonerated, his name was dragged through the mud and – to this day – even the most half-hearted Google search reveals a virtual footprint he can't escape. The nightmare was so traumatic he changed his name and left the country.

Yet, in spite of all this, nothing has been learned and all men remain at risk.

Oxford University students may be considered some of the most privileged young people in Britain, but Ben Sullivan – president of the university's 191-year-old debating society – didn't enjoy any such trappings when he was arrested at 6 a.m., detained for four hours in a police cell awaiting interview and publicly humiliated. He was just trapped.

For months he endured needless public suspicion before police sheepishly confirmed he wouldn't face a single charge. Not one. (Yet, for the privilege of it all, he still had to pay £15,000 in legal fees and, like Paul Weller or Bright Eyes singer Conor Oberst, have his life marred by a system that considers men's innocence a bonus, not a baseline.) As the allegations unfolded, Sarah Pine, President for Women at Oxford University's Student Union, spearheaded a campaign against him, even before the accusations were fully considered by police.

Typifying the way men are treated by so-called equality campaigners, she devised a boycott of scheduled guest speakers and called for Sullivan to resign. Interpol Secretary General Ronald Noble, Norman Finkelstein and – rather worryingly – David Mepham, UK Director of Human Rights Watch, all conceded. Only Jennifer Perry, CEO of the Digital Trust and author of the UK guidelines on digital risks, resisted – and later spoke of how she felt 'threatened' and 'intimidated' by Pine's gender-driven agenda.

An expert in cyber-stalking said she was subject to 'an enormous amount of pressure' by Pine, adding that she and her colleagues were asked 'in very forceful terms' to boycott Sullivan: 'It became apparent that [Pine's] agenda wasn't about keeping women safe and I don't want to be hijacked by someone else's political campaign. They are tramping on due process.'

Hence, when it was finally over, Sullivan earnestly

appeared across national media to defend a man's pre-conviction anonymity.

'An individual's identity should not automatically be revealed the minute they are arrested,' he said.

> There needs to be some happy medium where their identity is protected initially, until at least the conclusion of an investigation. These were utterly poisonous allegations against me. They were completely spurious, yet this was enough for an arrest. In cases like mine, everyone should have the right to anonymity as the inquiry is at a preliminary stage. The police and CPS should then be able to go to a judge and ask for the anonymity be waived, if they need it.
>
> I understand why naming people is useful, but when inquiries are at such an early stage it is vicious, and it can be at a huge cost.

Once again, this terrifying case in point not only proves that pre-conviction identification doesn't work, but re-iterates a very pertinent question: why, in our best ever age of equality, are men still being denied the right to a trial first? It's unjust and inhumane.

Originally, the law agreed. In 1976, the Labour government introduced rape trial anonymity for both the alleged victim and the accused. It operated this way until

1988, when guidelines were relaxed to help police investigations. At the time, the media was far less powerful, less global, less permanent than it is today. There was no internet, no slew of gossip magazines, no mobile phones with cameras, no social networking sites. Police techniques and technology were also less refined, so a lack of anonymity helped them.

Now, the landscape is different. Dramatically so. And – once again – the law should change to reflect this. Why? Because a not-guilty verdict is no longer enough to repair the planet-sized crater of damage caused by weeks of daily headlines across the globe.

Even Labour peer Lord Corbett, who introduced the 1976 law providing mutual pre-conviction anonymity, argued this until his death in February 2012. He told the *Evening Standard* in 2002: 'Rape is a uniquely serious offence and acquittal is not enough to clear a man in the eyes of his family, community or workplace. He is left with this indelible stain on his reputation. The case for matching anonymity for the defendant is as strong now as ever.'

He was right in life and he's right in death.

Maura McGowan, deputy High Court judge and chairwoman of the Bar Council, agrees. 'Until they have been proven to have done something as awful as this – I think there is a strong argument in cases of this sort, because they carry such stigma with them, to maintain the defendant's anonymity, until he is convicted,' she told BBC Radio 5.

> But once the defendant is convicted then of course everything should be open to scrutiny and to the public … [But] not all of these [rape] accusations are true and the damage that can be done to somebody's life … can be overwhelming if it isn't true. These cases are peculiar unto themselves because the stigma quite often can do so much damage.

One such case was that of Linsey Attridge. To stop her boyfriend leaving her, the 31-year-old claimed two men broke into her home and committed rape whilst he was away playing football. She then punched herself in the face and ripped her clothes to make the story appear credible, before spending three days trawling social networking sites to find users she could 'identify' as responsible. The men were then detained by police, questioned and forced to undergo intrusive forensic and medical examinations.

Two months later, Attridge confessed that it was a lie – but only received 200 hours of unpaid community service as punishment, which is neither a fitting penalty nor a deterrent.

Yet, for all their protestations about film storylines

and media representation, not one person or rape charity has ever come forward to denounce the culture of false allegations. Not one. They scold authors for writing books about women who lie about rape – *but won't get angry at the women who lie about rape*, which surely betrays real victims of rape more than pre-conviction anonymity ever could. Both the men and women who are attacked, and the men who are named and shamed regardless of conviction.

Sadly, it's not just real-life equivalents of *Gone Girl*'s Amy Dunne who deceive, but women in positions of power, too.

In 2010, an official inquiry report led by Baroness Stern – a prison reform campaigner – ordered Harriet Harman to stop misleading the public about rape statistics. For years she'd been pumping out misinformation that only 6 per cent of rapists are brought to justice, when the reality is very different. Actually, the 6 per cent figure relates to reported cases. *The conviction rate for those actually charged with rape is nearly two out of three, higher than comparable figures for other violent crime.*

A few weeks after Ben Sullivan's charges were dropped, I bumped into him in Soho – minutes after stumbling across MP Nigel Evans (who was similarly accused – then acquitted – of rape). Yet, whilst I vaguely recall a brief exchange with them both, what

I vividly remember is wondering if women like Harman or Bindel have ever seen men so ashen, so exhausted and so utterly violated by a system that's shaped by radical Marxist-based theories from the '70s. I doubt it.

Then again, even if they did, I suspect they'd dismiss such cases as profoundly exaggerated delusions of persecution. The suppression of dissident views is saddening.

Yet, what conversely makes me smile about the politics around *Gone Girl* and its difficult subject matter is that the framework for response is strikingly similar to that of anti-Thatcherism. After all, one of the reasons Britain's only female Prime Minister remains so passionately hated is that, like Rosamund Pike's character, she revealed a damning secret about women which ruins their image – that they can be just as vile, just as evil, just as dangerous as men.

It's as if these people make the issue about men v. women, rather than right v. wrong, which is both the epitome of those man-hating feminist clichés and, crucially, a dead-end path to justice – especially when rape victims can be of either gender. Statistics from America's National Crime Victimisation Survey recently revealed 38 per cent of rape survivors in a 40,000 sample were men, whilst records from the Bureau of Justice Statistics noted half of these men reported a female attacker.

Besides, the benefit of mutual anonymity would serve

all, helping victims as well as conserving fair trials. For a start, it would deter anyone from making false claims out of spite, potentially seeing the accuracy of convictions rise – not fall. Secondly, it could make testifying easier for those who've come forward. Identifying the accused often inadvertently identifies the victim, which adds immense pressure for them. It's all wrong.

This is common sense, but it's also the view of the majority. When the subject was mooted in a poll on – funnily enough – the *Guardian* website, 71 per cent of readers supported pre-conviction anonymity. A similar survey by MailOnline showed that 67 per cent of readers feel the same.

The consensus is clear: in a world of grey areas, consent is always black and white – but the protection of anonymity must be too.

THE REAL MEN'S HEALTH

THE TRUTH HURTS – BUT NO more than terminal cancer, sudden cardiac arrest or having one of your testicles surgically removed. You may want to remember this as you read the following chapter, because, although it isn't typically feel-good stuff, it'll also certainly feel better than each of the above – and might just save your life.

According to the Office for National Statistics, men don't just lead in nine of the top ten killer diseases, including cancer, heart disease, stroke, pneumonia, diabetes and cirrhosis of the liver – you know, the really fun ones – we also die five years earlier than women in a life expectancy gap that's increased 400 per cent since 1920.

This alone should be the klaxon-sounding wake-up call we need to storm Parliament and start a protest – or, at the very least, a hashtag. Then again, given the amount of well-being warnings we're bombarded with on a daily basis – smoking kills, drugs are bad, eat five a day, mind the gap, caution: filling is hot – we can be forgiven for lazy reflexes. It's a bit like the emergency evacuation procedure on a plane: yeah, yeah, we know – let's just get going and we'll cross that bridge when we come to it. Except, whilst aeronautical disasters are pretty rare, our own crash landings are inevitable. In fact, we're dropping like flies.

We are, dare I say it, the Malaysian Airlines of the genders.

Which is exactly why the following pages square up to a fear most human beings are exceptionally skilful at ignoring: the nagging reality that, from the moment we are born into life, the clock is ticking. From the sound of the starting gun, death appears over the horizon and is racing towards us faster than a drunk driver in a double-decker. The crucial bit nobody dares address – which is why it needs an entire chapter here, part-written in big shouty capital letters – is that, in the ugliness of dog-eat-dog survival, it's men, not women, who are thrown under the bus.

A report by the Bureau of Investigative Journalism found that 'in almost two-thirds of London's wards, the gap between men and women's life expectancy is wider than the national average of 4.1 years'. In the city's more deprived parts, 'women outlive men by more than twelve years … That's worse than Russia, the country where, relatively, men live the world's second-shortest lives compared to their female counterparts.' A fact backed up by the World Health Organization.

Forensically, the BIJ report noted that, between 2007 and 2012, NHS Primary Care Trusts in the capital's Haringey, Hammersmith & Fulham, Brent and Camden 'spent a total of £4,830,095 commissioning women's services outside the NHS over the past five years, and nothing on men's' – a trend which is visible nationally, with female care almost constantly ranked above men's.

The ultimate insult? It's all done at our expense – literally and metaphorically. The National Health Service is funded by the public purse, but it's men – yes, men; you know, the hairy ones on the gurneys – who pay a whopping 70 per cent of UK income tax. Just ask the Queen. A Freedom of Information Act request to Her Majesty's Revenue & Customs revealed that men coughed up 71.2 per cent of it for 2010/11, yet were thrown crumbs in return.

The people at the top know this and have done for

ages. Fifteen years ago the UK's Men's Health Forum published stats that, for every £1 spent on men's health, £8 was spent on women's – but since then little has changed for no good reason. Or, rather, one very *bad* reason: we live in a medical matriarchy.

In other words, male life is cheap. Primark cheap.

Sadly, this isn't just a domestic issue. Data gathered from Australia's National Health and Medical Research Council – the body which allocates all government funding Down Under – recently found a 'spectacular gender gap', with 'men's health problems being allocated a quarter of the funding women's research gets'. In fact, men's health ranked thirty-sixth, 'behind sexually transmitted infections and just ahead of parasitic infections'.

Stateside, Barack Obama may have promised change, but what he's actually proposing is short change. The Affordable Care Act is littered with random inequities for men. Browse through it and you'll find 134 references to women's health – great – but just two for ours, and even then they're fleeting. You'll find an entire chapter dedicated to breast cancer, yet prostate cancer isn't even mentioned.

Forget the American dream, this is a bloody nightmare.

'I wrote in *Time* magazine that women should pay more for ObamaCare because they get more, which is fair, but I've never seen such a vitriolic response,' says Hadley

Heath, a senior policy analyst specialising in health, economics and fiscal policy at the Independent Women's Forum in New York. 'There was real abuse for the suggestion that men shouldn't bankroll women's healthcare, but then I realised it's not about being fair, it's about giving women a good deal at any cost – even if that cost is men's lives.'

Like I said, the truth hurts. But, according to Gloria Steinem, it can also set you free – well, once it's pissed you off. What pisses me off, however, is that rather than being the subject of sympathetic public concern or the odd fundraising gala, men are just repeatedly told it's all their fault. Every day, some self-appointed expert lays the responsibility for our government-endorsed premature deaths on 'the narrow definitions of masculinity', as if The Rock himself is sat there divvying up healthcare funding.

This is bollocks.

Men aren't dying sooner because they're ignorant or proud – it's because the entire system leaves them to rot and, politically, they're discouraged from doing anything about it. After all, that would be sexist.

Don't buy any other excuse, ever. In fact, look at what we *do* buy. Trends in print media blow this ignoramus excuse out of the water. Sneak a peek into any man's house and, right there – in the ironically named living room – is a stack of *Men's Health* magazines, our biggest-selling monthly, with twelve million readers. Fine, after a few cursory, laconic glances they're left to gather dust at the side of the sofa – suggesting the mere presence of a six-pack increases the likelihood of us getting one by sheer proximity alone. As if it's contagious, like Ebola. But who cares? They still double up as glossy pieces of proof that the first step to good health – the desire to live long and prosper, as Mr Spock asserted – is already within us.

'Men's relative lack of self-care compared to women is a contributing factor to their shorter life expectancy, but only a *very minor* one,' says Dr Timothy Spector, a Professor of Genetic Epidemiology at King's College.

> Compared to women, men have shorter markers of longevity, called telomeres – suggesting there'll always be a biological difference [which justifies the need for men to get greater care]. The state needs to realise that they are discriminated against by the set-up of the current UK system.

Indeed.

This, rather appropriately, shifts the blame back onto the people who deserve it – the big cheeses who make all these *Titanic*-era women-and-children-first decisions for us. The same experts who are personally responsible for making men 25 per cent more likely to suffer one of the 152,000 strokes in Britain each year, for example.

OK, fine, there's no incriminating paper trail to say they're directly to blame – no chain of emails we can present to an official inquiry – but only because there needn't be. Rather than expending precious energy creating our downfall, the architects of this fatal structure – usually armed with private healthcare, I might add – know they can get exactly the same results by doing nothing at all. 'Let them eat cake!' they say, fully aware the fat will eventually collect around our middle and block our arteries, rendering us a few million fewer to worry about. Job done.

I know, I know. It's bleak stuff and I sound like a cranky conspiracy theorist, but – hey – at least I call a spade a spade. If we apply the Alcoholics Anonymous theory of recovery to improving men's health, the first step is admitting a problem exists in the first place. So it's funny that when men do die – even, say, as civilian casualties in a bomb explosion where it's *definitely* not their fault – they vanish from the English language. Newsreaders with Oxford educations suddenly develop a Gareth Gates-style stutter with the word 'm-m-m-m-men' and report that 'Two hundred people died this afternoon – including seventy-four women and three children.' Oh, right. And who were the others? Extras from *The Muppet Show*?

Rather than object to this and say 'Oi! Matriarchy

– NO!', we've realised it's much easier to name just one man and grieve for him specifically. This is allowed (for now).

I write these words on the same day Rik Mayall dies of a massive, sudden heart attack. The comedian was just fifty-six when it happened – not old by any stretch of the imagination. On the contrary, fifty-six doesn't just *seem* young these days, it *is* young. As the life expectancy goes up, the mean age for what's youthful also increases. But he didn't just have age on his side. The *Young Ones* star was also actively looking after himself; he collapsed following his routine morning run.

Naturally, everybody shared their sympathy. 'What a waste! So sad! Life's unfair!' But in recognition of all the out-pouring, his wife said: 'I'm sure you all know Rik's response would be something along the lines of: "Well, thanks very much all of you ... now fuck off!"', which was perfectly fitting because, without his household name status, Rik Mayall would've been just one of the 200 people who die of heart disease each day; the majority of whom are men. That's 73,000 each year.

Still, there's absolutely no sense of urgency about stemming this constant, preventable loss. On the contrary, people panic about cellulite instead.

OK, I'm tub-thumping, but perhaps I need to in order to be heard over the huge vortex of crap thinking which goes hand-in-hand with men's health. Not only aren't we immunised, funded properly, debated or treated equally to women, we also aren't given the same empathy as them. When former Deputy Prime Minister John Prescott revealed he had bulimia, the world laughed. Yes, eating disorders are funny! Who knew!

The Sun declared his condition a misdiagnosis, saying: 'He 'wasn't a very successful bulimic. As in so many other areas of life, not very successful at all.' Meanwhile, the ever-moralistic and equality-conscious Jezebel produced a 'What Prezza Was Eating … Daily Guidelines for Men' – complete with fat and carbohydrate content – which showed others how to develop the illness. They also binged on the idea that 'men can really make an achievement out of this shit', whilst insinuating fathers were to blame.

Well, I'll be damned: the feminists at Jezebel are sexist.

But at least they prove a point. After all, would women be spoken about like this? Would it be tolerated? No way. Which is a whole other killer malaise: the fact that men still aren't allowed to be weak on their own terms. Just look how TV adverts for high street pharmacies constantly show women multi-tasking through stage four leukemia, whilst men go to bed with a sore throat. The subtext is that women are stoic heroines, whilst men who get sick are wimps.

When men don't discuss their health concerns it's not because they're wired this way, it's because they're responding to social codes of behaviour. After all, if they say anything they'll be greeted with shaming tactics to stop them. Look at something as brilliant as Movember. It has been a global success and saved countless lives, yet journalist Arianne Shavisi wrote in the *New Statesman* that 'Movember is divisive, gender normative, racist and ineffective'.

Her precise gripe was that Movember is really about 'white young men ridiculing minorities', whilst being 'sexist' and celebrating 'imperialism'. Dispensing more pearls of wisdom, she added that it was inherently misogynistic because women can't grow facial hair. Now, perhaps she hasn't used the London Underground at rush hour, or wasted an afternoon in Stoke Newington, but that's definitely not true. Besides, not every single action has to be extended to the opposite sex. We are equal, but different. One approach doesn't always fit all.

Regardless of this, she insisted it's women who are suffering, not the men shitting themselves because they've been diagnosed with cancer and might die. 'In solidarity with Movember, some women have also relaxed normative shaving-etiquette ... [but] instead of being met with the same teasing words of encouragement ... [we learn that] female breaches of prescribed gender norms are quickly policed, and may result in disgust,' she added. 'Movember is a reminder that women should think carefully before subverting their sexually objectified bodies to join in with boy's games.'

Fortunately, what resulted was a hilarious stream of faith-restoring, common-sense clarity in the comments section.

One reader responded:

> Oh, you're quite right. As a woman, I've always regretted my inability to grow facial hair, whilst my husband can achieve a full beard in a month if and when he can't be bothered to shave. So long have I been oppressed. But no more. This article has encouraged me to take up the fight and ensure that no man, regardless of race or religion, can ever grow facial hair again until all women are able to do so. I want a hairy upper lip but if I can't have one, I'm going to make sure that none of them can! Who cares if it's a natural biological process, when society is in danger of toppling due to their selfish desire to have hairy faces? Alternatively this article is a pile of utter tripe and the author really needs to chill out a bit.

Another wrote: 'Burst out laughing at the first mention of the word "racist", then, as I realised you were serious, I felt a kind of astonished pity.'

Personally, my favourite was simply: 'I. WANT. TO. CRY. This is why we can't have nice things.'

Turn on the TV for light relief and you'll see the same thing, but in a different guise. When Steve in HBO's *Sex and the City* got testicular cancer it was, according to the scriptwriters, comedy gold. We had Kim Cattrall's alter ego leaning over a snooker table with a cue, saying she only had 'one ball left to pot', which was charming. I know when I'm stuck sucking on a Milk Maid – the iced lolly, not an actual farm girl – in a chemotherapy unit trying to fight testicular cancer, I'll hold onto this clip and gain strength. Yet, when the same character gets breast cancer, she suddenly turns into Stephen Sutton, who, I might add, was anything but the typical weak man as he looked death straight in the eye, full of dignity, and raised £4 million for charity, bagging himself a posthumous MBE too.

Then, of course, there's the whole double standard of fitness as sexual appeal.

Only recently there was a Victoria's Secret advert which sparked 'outrage' because all its models were lithe and toned. Critics photoshopped bigger, alternative bodies onto the ad and created a meme. Then there's the Dove 'Real Women' campaign which sees plus-sized, shapely sisters lining up to show off their rounder bodies as proof of big beauty.

But can you imagine if men did the same? Let's say we make a similar response to the David Gandy underwear posters for Marks & Spencer – complete with men in pants showing off their beer bellies, bald spots and ingrown hairs with the strapline 'This Is What Real Men Look Like' – there'd be all the typical hatred and resistance. Yet, whilst women have anorexia and bulimia, guess what – so do men. They also have an entire sub-culture of 'bigorexia' which sees them pump their bodies with steroids and protein shakes because all they're ever told is that bulge size matters – not just in the trousers or the wallet, but in the arms and chest too.

Still, columnists would fall over themselves to say how ugly the male body is or point to the images as proof of what horrors women 'suffer' in the bedroom. Actually, the opposite is true.

See, whilst we're on the subject of sex, it turns out that going down on Catherine Zeta-Jones might kill us, too. Is *nothing* sacred? When actor Michael Douglas announced his battle with throat cancer was caused by oral sex – or, more specifically, the HPV virus contracted through oral sex – he made a nation of men gulp at the realisation they're living with a ticking timebomb. The 69-year-old, who fought a six-month battle with the disease, said: 'Without wanting to get too specific, this particular cancer is caused by HPV, which comes about from cunnilingus.'

Currently, girls aged twelve and thirteen are routinely vaccinated against the virus because of its link to cervical cancer. They also receive a top-up injection at eighteen. But for men, there's no effective screening test and no NHS immunisation.

We might shrug our shoulders to this, but cases of oral cancer have risen by 50 per cent among UK men since 1989 and now account for almost 2,000 deaths per year. HPV infections also remain common in men as they get older, whereas it tends to become less prevalent in their female counterparts. This may be because men are less likely than women to develop immunity, even after repeated exposure. Additional research conducted by scientists at the Cancer Centre and Research Institute in Florida found those with fifty or more sexual partners were 2.4 times more likely to develop cancer than those with just one.

Worried? You should be. I call Macmillan Cancer Support and hope they'll play it down, but they don't. They can't. 'We know the number of oral cancers related to the HPV virus in men is rising, so it is important to take this seriously,' says Dr Rosie Loftus, the charity's lead GP advisor.

At the moment, parents have to seek private treatment, which can cost £150, if they would like their son to be vaccinated [before they start having oral sex], whilst it is free for girls on the NHS. Everyone, regardless of gender, age or where they live in the UK, should get access to the best possible treatment.

Unsurprisingly, the wider issue of cancer is no more morale-boosting. Currently, women are screened for breast cancer, ovarian and cervical cancer – which, again, is great – but excuse me if I don't jump up and down. It's either a) the weight of my male privilege or b) the sobering reality that there's *still* no screening programme for prostate cancer, even though we know it kills four times more men than cervical cancer does women. In fact, experts predict that in twenty years' time prostate cancer will be the most common form of the disease – which is alarming considering only half the population have prostates.

Don't be too shocked by this. Research compiled by Cancer Research UK illustrates that men are 16 per cent more likely to develop every single form of unisex cancer in the first place, then 40 per cent more likely to die from it. Despite this, their Race for Life fundraiser bans men and boys from participating every year – just because they're male and, presumably, might put poles in the grass and expect all the lady runners to dance around them, gyrating and pouting for their entertainment.

BECAUSE ALL MEN DO THIS, ALL THE TIME, AND NO MEN EVER WANT TO SIMPLY FUN-DRAISE FOR CANCER WITHOUT BECOMING HYPNOTISED BY THE SEXUAL POWER OF WOMEN AND OBJECTIFY THEM.

'Three years ago, we seriously investigated the possibility of including men in Race for Life,' they told me. 'However, our research showed that our supporters would strongly prefer to keep it a female-only event as it's a unique opportunity for women to come together in a non-competitive activity within an atmosphere of sisterhood.'

Ah, I see. So forget that men are universally dying from cancer more frequently, and faster, than women. Instead, we should worry about keeping the texture of a global disease 'special' to reserve a charity's USP. To be fair, I'm sure teenage boys who've lost their mother to cancer love nothing more than double-glazing the glass ceiling whilst 500 women in New Look leggings walk, briefly jog, immediately slow down to a canter, then walk again, in a field on a wet Sunday.

Somebody book me a fucking room in Dignitas before this madness gets any worse.

Naturally, I see their point – they don't want to change a winning formula. But *my* point is that it's only a winning formula if you're a woman, which – by the very principle of equality – means it's NOT a winning formula.

Being realistic, it's us men who have long been making the rules, so, if inconsistencies have been put in place, it's likely we shot ourselves in the foot. But, at the same time, we've long had a grip on equality, with plenty of powerful women making decisions too, so all this could've ironed out by now. Instead, there isn't one person in government who's responsible for improving men's health. Not one.

This, you might say, is a total pisser. Not least because another toss of the dice and it could be me. My father had cancer, as did my mother. With the exception of some love handles, I'm pretty much in shape according to BMI standards, but let's be honest: I drink a bit too much, occasionally smoke and have a typical journalist's diet (box wine and canapés). Given my family history and my lifestyle combined, chances are I'll also develop the Big C. On one hand, I can deal with this prospect – it's the Russian roulette of life. Everybody gets something. But what I absolutely can't resolve – and I've tried – is that I'm much, much, much more likely to die for the simple reason that men aren't politically fashionable.

One person who experienced this first-hand was my Uncle Al.

Back in the early '60s, he was already a Suffragent. Yes, he forever had girlfriends, but he also made it clear that he'd never marry because, quite simply, he enjoyed his freedom and marriage was a con. He also didn't casually spawn children – never had any, by choice, and managed this carefully. Ultimately, he was faithful to himself, which is the cornerstone of any manhood-standing bloke.

That said, he was also a *Carry On* character in our very own family. First there was the time he worked as an accounts clerk at the Bird's Eye factory in Liverpool during the 1970s and, spotting a woman he regularly played practical jokes with, grabbed her by the ankles and tipped her into the 5ft-deep freezer she was browsing – only to realise it was somebody else. Then there was the day he went commando in a pair of light-green summer trousers to the office, only to be told by a neighbour on his way home that they were see-through. Or the time he was asked to completely undress for a medical and 'get on the examination bed', only for the doctor to return some time later – after various nurses had been in and out – and urge: 'Mr McCracken, I meant *under* the sheets.'

By 2007, when commerce in Liverpool picked up, he worked for a firm in the Cunard Building – one of the city's three architectural graces alongside the famous Liver Birds. As he approached a well-earned and comfortable retirement, having worked all his life, he started complaining of stomach pains. IBS, we casually diagnosed. Maybe an ulcer. Too much food?

For months he went to his doctor's as the pain

worsened and his weight plummeted, but, in the midst of a busy GP surgery packed with women and children, I can only assume he didn't stand out as being particularly important. Over time, his doctor failed to order the right tests. Even when she did, she lost the results. She later promised to make a referral to a specialist, but forgot. On one occasion she called him in for his appointment by the wrong name as she clutched another man's file, even though he was now a regular. Together, this all conspired to create the perfect storm which meant his bowel cancer was left undetected for so long it had spread.

Six weeks later he was dead.

That was in 2009, but even now, years on, I wonder: what more could've been done to save him? Did the fact he was a man make him fall to the back of the queue? Sounds like typical loss speaking, yes, but if the statistics show we die at higher rates and at younger ages than women, and that funding for male care is often non-existent – meaning we're invisible on paper – why wouldn't plenty of men be killed by inadvertent discrimination as a consequence? And, if I'm right, should we be worried as the NHS becomes increasingly female?

Two years ago I caused a storm when I sued my local gym for hosting a women's hour – in part, to get beyond the media veil on men's issues. Specifically, I objected to the sports centre banning men and boys for 442 hours each year – despite charging them the same annual fee as women. I suggested they change their policy with one of three alternatives: a) maintain a women's hour but introduce a men's alternative for fairness, b) keep women's hour (and only women's hour) but annually charge men less, or c) scrap single-gender sessions altogether.

They declined. Their justification? Lots of women feel bad about their bodies – and, essentially, all men are perverts, so I should suck it up.

This ridiculous ruling simply proved my theory that everyone is looking at the wrong end of the telescope. Actually, it's *men* who need more assistance getting into gyms – not women. Why? Because the physical pressure on them, working full-time, combined with all of the above, actively contributes to our shorter life expectancy.

One reason women live longer is because, among other things, they have more choices: chances to shift gear or change lanes. The opportunity to opt out of the rat race at any time. They can be career women, work in PR until they get married, or be a lady who lunches. Perhaps a combination of all three. Generally, men need to be self-reliant always, all the time, forever. Increased fitness offsets this.

In Augusten Burrough's *Running with Scissors*, he talks about playing 'Bible Dip' in his youth – an act of divination he likens to asking a Magic 8 Ball a question, only to God. For the response, he would open the Bible at a random page and whatever word his finger landed on was the answer. I apply this approach to the nearest copy of *Healthy for Men* which my Dad, now seventy, reads whilst eating half a pack of biscuits. Even though he's diabetic since his cancer treatment.

I audibly ask it: 'Aside from the aforementioned, what is the big, unspoken men's health issue of the moment?' And let the pages fall. The results are less biblical, more typical. First there's 'Pack a Pork Lunch', which presents the virtues of a protein-heavy diet, followed by a feature on how to build last-minute, pre-holiday muscle (which I rip out and keep, but never read), then a briefing on the benefits of Vitamin D. All pedestrian stuff, really.

Dispirited, I give it one last go – and am momentarily stunned into stillness. Fuck! I cannot quite believe it. There's a feature on male suicide. Contained in a magazine. About men's health. It's almost *logical*.

The people behind it are from CALM, the Campaign Against Living Miserably, who've fought tooth and nail to break into the public consciousness with the real men's health, forcing us onto the agenda in the face of resistance.

'Don't be fooled. Many organisations have a vested interest in ignoring men,' says Jane Powell, the charity's dynamic director.

When CALM was launched as a pilot by the Department of Health in 2006, we got £30,000 because they had to be seen to be doing something to stop the rates of men killing themselves – but we haven't had a penny from them since. They did the minimum.

When I recently applied for a government grant, all the tick-boxes were for women or minorities. There was nothing, at all, just for men. So when I asked if I could use the 'hard to reach' group for them, they said no – that it would be sexist. But what other distinguishing characteristics did they want for male suicide? The most common factor is their gender. What part of men being 77 per cent of cases did they not understand?

Finally! Some sense. And it couldn't have come at a better time – our suicide rates are at a ten-year high and show no signs of slowing down. In 2012, there were 5,981 cases, of which 4,590 were male.

Unfortunately, this alone means it's not worthy of mainstream attention.

'If we were talking about women it'd be a piece of piss – we'd have high-profile celebrity supporters and slots on breakfast TV. The media would relish it,' she adds.

But there's always been a reluctance to discuss gender and suicide. Only now, in the latest strategy report, has it finally been referred to as *male* suicide, rather than *young* suicide – and even then it skips over it. People actually say to me: 'We can't talk about this because it will upset feminists.' And I'm a feminist!

It's incredibly frustrating. The women's movement has had a huge positive impact on society, but we've also colonised the debate on everything. In doing so, there's never been any space for men to respond – and that's clearly very destructive. As a proud feminist, it's crucial that everyone has a fair chance. Feminism – and feminists – must start talking about the needs and rights of men and boys too. Otherwise, at what point do we start giving men permission to be men? And who the hell are we to take it from them?

The question is a pertinent one, because that's exactly what this is all about men: the freedom to have a healthy approach to health, without smears and slurs of sexism.

Essentially, like a game of Bible Dip, the answer already exists somewhere in the mix. To use it, what we need is a brand-new NHS body with a heart that beats to the sound of reality's drum – not the fist-thumping of political games.

BIGMOUTHS
STRIKE AGAIN

RUBY WAX ONCE TOLD ME fame is a disease – and that, back in her TV heyday, she would interview celebrities to see how severely they had it.

Ever since then I've imagined it to be like the Zika virus. Except, rather than shrinking babies' heads, this particular contagion causes the egos of light entertainers to swell irreversibly. Imagine *28 Days Later* played out in

Soho House or the Groucho Club, with the condition characterised by an inability to entertain without voicing unsolicited opinions on everything from the Schengen Agreement to NAFTA.

Recent offenders include Benedict Cumberbatch, who patronised theatre-goers on behalf of Syrian refugees, despite the fact that he still won't share his massive house with any, er, Syrian refugees; luvvie actress Emma Thompson (a staunch socialist – if you overlook the fact that she's thunderingly posh and sent her daughter to private school); and, of course, Lady Gaga, who co-wrote the song 'Til It Happens to You' for *The Hunting Ground*, a documentary suggesting that Ivy League college campuses are overrun with rapists (except, er, they're not).

These instant politicos – just add water and stir! – have little substance, even less insight and scant regard for what audiences actually want from them.

This is particularly naff when it comes to the never-ending gender debate, where a catalogue of crashing bores seek easy sainthood by delivering factually incorrect sermons on the sisterhood.

So, to remedy this cancer – and its humourless tumours – the following serves as a bitter pill/debrief/open letter for those who, when it comes to hectoring, should rather keep their mouths shut.

EMMA WATSON

Given that she's endorsed skin-whitening creams, you wouldn't think Emma Watson needed to lighten up – but, trust me, she does. Despite being one of the world's most accomplished and upper-class stars, she still moans about being a victim. Which, to be fair, she is – OF DELUSION.

One of her favourite gripes is that all men are always privileged all of the time, whilst all women are always oppressed all of the time. Yet her very own lived experience contradicts this.

Born in Paris to lawyer parents, she attended Oxford's ultra-posh Dragon School, which – FYI – costs £9,340 per term. After this, she enrolled at Headington Girls' School, which kindly relieves attendees of £10,300 every semester.

Since then she's amassed a £48 million fortune, according to the *Sunday Times Rich List*, which is good for her – but it's also more than 90 per cent of men will earn in a lifetime.

Yet, despite this, she continues to bang on about her hard-knock life as if this is *Annie: The Musical*.

Publicly playing out her struggle at every available opportunity, she surpassed herself recently when she received journalistic cunnilingus from *Esquire* for what can only be described as their cuckold issue. Telling men (via a brow-beaten Tom Hanks), 'This isn't your fault – but it is your problem,' she patronised readers by quoting Martin Luther King and saying blokes should 'talk about their feelings', be less dominant and 'listen to their girlfriends'.

OH, FUCK OFF!

Let's keep it real here: firstly, men aren't stupid and don't need a masterclass in equality from some 25-year-old. Secondly, if men do talk about their feelings, or cry, they're usually ridiculed by women who a) declare them wimps, then b) tell them to 'man up', which is a phrase Watson herself admits using.

In fact, only a few years ago, she said she'd never date a British man again because they were too unassertive. 'English guys are very restrained,' she complained. Whereas American men would be brash and say something akin to 'get your coat, you've pulled', which she confessed to finding more attractive.

Make your mind up, love.

Then again, this type of double standard is nothing new to Watson. After lecturing her 21 million Twitter followers about how men were 'imprisoned by gender stereotypes' of machismo, she quickly dated muscle-man rugby player and 'Oxford's most eligible bachelor' Matthew Janney. Twelve months later, she reportedly hooked up with the equally strapping William Knight, a tech entrepreneur and marathon-running gym-bunny.

Seeing a pattern, much? No beta males here.

Hilariously, when the *Daily Mail* acknowledged this contradiction in an article entitled 'Hermione the Hypocrite', she got uppity via her lawyers, who made a (rather measly) defence on her behalf.

Which is ironic considering she's supposedly strong and independent.

MADONNA

Once the behemoth talent who defined female success in the '80s, Madonna – like so many other women – has now fallen foul of her own female privilege concerning motherhood, suggesting that even pop culture's most powerful female force indulges in gender inequality when it suits.

Those with an internet connection will know that she threw her toys out of the pram when fifteen-year-old son Rocco chose to live with his father, Guy Ritchie, over her.

Vexed by the dent to her ego, she swiftly filed kidnapping charges with a federal judge in Manhattan (even though the kid went of his own volition) and continued to vent her spleen at unsuspecting theatre-goers worldwide.

To be fair, I do sympathise – but not too much, because men have been dealing with this shit for years. In fact, poor Guy himself missed most of his son's childhood because Madge decided to relocate Rocco to the USA, so she should consider herself lucky.

She should also write the words 'I MADE MY BED SO I WILL LIE IN IT' on Post-it notes and attach them to mirrors throughout her home. Why? Because it's true. She's the one who moved him abroad – thousands of miles away from his father. The only reason she's annoyed now is because it backfired and she doesn't like the taste of her own medicine.

Like so many others, she should remember that her child is theirs, not hers.

PATRICIA ARQUETTE

She's starred in *True Romance* and *Boyhood*, which suggests an impressive knack for picking good projects, but poor ol' Patty is less successful when it comes to identifying fact from feminist guff.

Everyone knows she delivered a patronising lecture on alleged Hollywood pay inequality during the Oscars, but one look at this woman's Twitter timeline shows she rarely discusses anything else. In fact, her entire conversational repertoire seems to be built on Sandi Toksvig's political manifesto.

Even when I met her at the BAFTAs, where you'd think she'd actually be having a night off from saving the world, she spent the entire time asserting how oppressed she was whilst simultaneously clutching the Best Actress gong. Seriously, how oppressed can she be if she's reaching the top of her game?

Some time later, when the Kesha/Sony Records case was thrown out by a judge in April 2016 (the singer wanted to be released from her contract with music producer Dr Luke after she claimed he raped her – something he strenuously denies and she has never pressed charges over), Patricia posted online: 'Please remove that judge from the bench. He needs mental health treatment' – which is unfortunate considering it was actually a woman called Justice Shirley Werner Kornreich.

This might not seem like a biggie, but it suggests she's one of the many fainting-couch feminists whose default response to everything is that it's men subjugating women, which smacks of a victim complex.

She later added: '[Rape] law in itself is discriminatory & written through a lense [*sic*] of biased gender discrimination.' And, interestingly, she's right – although not in the way she thinks, because thanks to the women's movement, rape is legally defined so it can only be perpetrated by a man. Hence 35-year-old female teachers who sleep with twelve-year-old boys are frequently only charged with 'sexual assault', not statutory rape.

Oh, and whilst we're at it, she might also want to revisit the Change.org petition she started, which makes the bananas claim that 'the United States does not adequately protect women's human rights'.

Excuse me? I'm sure they still have issues like any other social group, but American women are some of the most privileged people on the planet. Moreover, there is no war being waged against them.

Fellow actress Jodie Foster recently nailed it when she said at the Tribeca Film Festival: 'I'm a little sick of talking about the woman thing. I don't think there is a big plot to keep women down.'

Amen.

HELEN MIRREN

Opinions are like arseholes – everyone's got one, but we all think everyone else's stinks.

This rather crude analogy needs to be shared with Helen Mirren, because she's a classic example of someone who believes her own hype, then develops a messiah complex and rams her ire down our throats – regardless of enthusiastic consent.

Speaking in the *Mail on Sunday*'s *You* magazine, she recently chided 'sexist' men who had the temerity to – brace yourselves – put their arm around a girlfriend. Explaining herself, she mused:

> If I could give my younger self one piece of advice, it would be to use the words 'fuck off' much more frequently. It annoys me when I see men with an arm slung round a woman's shoulders. It's like ownership. When I see girls being leaned on, I want to say, 'Tell him to get his damned arm off your shoulder.'

First of all, a quick Google image search confirms what I already suspected: that she either needs to practise what she preaches – or at least get her manager to remove the countless pictures of her draped all over poor husband Taylor Hackford, which ever-so-slightly undermine her argument.

Secondly, her suggestion is totally ludicrous. Does this mean gay men who put an arm around their partner are also being oppressive – rather than romantically expressive? What about lesbians who do the same with girlfriends? And straight women with men?

It's called romance, FFS.

BENEDICT CUMBERBATCH

When he's not directing the resolution of Europe's migrant crisis from his ivory tower, Benedict loves to get all serious and address the really big, urgent issues facing women – namely, the jokey moniker 'Cumberbitch'.

Rather than a bit of innocent wordplay his female fans used to describe themselves, he educated humanity (through an interview with Caitlin Moran for *The Times*, of course) that it was living proof of systematic misogyny. Who knew?

'I won't allow you to be my bitches,' he said, smugly. 'I think it sets feminism back so many notches. You are … Cumberpeople.'

VOMITS IN MOUTH

In case his loyalty to the cause wasn't clear, he later took a break from calling black people 'coloured' (cringe) and posed in a T-shirt stating 'This is What a Feminist Looks Like' – you know, the ones sold for £45, but produced for 62p an hour via the exploitation of women in Mauritian sweatshops. The same women who sleep sixteen to a room and told the *Mail on Sunday*'s investigative reporter: 'We don't feel like feminists. We don't feel equal. We feel trapped.'

Because, in case you didn't get the memo, the plight of modern oppression is primarily suffered by free, educated, autonomous women who watch BBC productions of Sherlock Holmes on sofas from Dwell.

Bore off, Benedict.

SARAH SILVERMAN

Like so many of her contemporaries, comedian Sarah Silverman is determined (or, rather, desperate) to be oppressed.

Specifically, she claims to pay a 'vagina tax', which – instead of being invoiced by the IRS – I assume is secretly deducted by the patriarchy, because she's never been able to substantiate it.

In fact, continuing that time-honoured feminist tradition, she went one better and deliberately lied through her teeth about it.

Recording a campaign video for Levo League women's organisation (nope, I'd not heard of them either), Silverman claimed she was paid $10 for a live appearance at the New York Comedy Club, whilst her male co-star received $60 – just for being a bloke. Ooh.

Naturally, this was received with glee by media feminists – until the venue's owner, Al Martin, heard the libellous claim and publicly clarified that she was full of shit.

He replied on social media, saying:

> Are you kidding? You came into my club 15 years ago and asked me for a guest spot. I did not ask you to perform and you were not booked. Then you ask me for pay?
>
> I did not pay you less cause of gender … I paid you less because Todd Barry was booked and you weren't. It was a GUEST SPOT, so I gave you some car fare, which actually is more than almost any club would have given for a GUEST Spot. Funny how in your attempt to become a super hero with a noble cause, you forgot that little fact … GUEST SPOT … GUEST SPOT.

I don't know about you, but that's the best laugh I've had in ages.

ASHTON KUTCHER

The former flame of Demi Moore scored brownie points when he took to Twitter demanding that men's public bathrooms have an equal number of baby-changing facilities to women's.

Seriously, Ashton, this should NOT be your biggest concern in the fatherhood debate. Besides, MOST

MEN'S TOILETS DON'T HAVE BABY-CHANGING FACILITIES BECAUSE MANY MEN DON'T HAVE ACCESS TO THEIR BABIES. I've written an entire chapter on the matter. Read it and see for yourself.

But, that said, if you're so bothered about restroom amenities, then get yourself down to the M&S in Angel, because they have them – and have done for years. They're also well-used, which goes to show how hands-on the men of Islington are.

In the meantime, maybe you can get equally vociferous about, say, the issues of paternity fraud or shared parenting? Give Guy Ritchie a call. He can fill you in.

LENA DUNHAM

Christ, I don't even know where to start with this wretch. Actually, yes, I do – the false rape claim in her ironically titled book *Not That Kind of Girl*.

Keen to paint herself as some sort of victim/heroine, the *Girls* actress (read: well-connected Manhattan brat who had doors opened by Daddy) claimed she'd been raped at Oberlin College by a prominent campus Republican named Barry, who worked in the library and was a student in her peer group.

In other words, she implicated him by everything but name.

Unsurprisingly, this poor, easily identifiable bloke – who was a family man when this went down – became the subject of intense media scrutiny and was forced to hire a defence lawyer, Aaron Minc, who issued a statement of innocence via the *National Review*.

It was only when Breitbart News published a lengthy investigative report (which eventually cleared him) that Dunham and her publishers, Random House, finally admitted it was all fake. Except, by this point, Dunham had known of this innocent man's turmoil for FOUR WHOLE MONTHS AND DID NOTHING ABOUT IT.

Referencing this minor matter, Minc said:

> We were gratified to find out that Random House 'regrets the confusion' about Lena Dunham's false accusation. We also welcome Random House's offer to pay legal expenses.
>
> However, we remain disappointed and troubled for the following reasons: We have been contacting Random House and Ms. Dunham, seeking an apology and exoneration. Our repeated pleas to handle this quietly and with dignity were met with indifference. It wasn't until more than $20,000 was raised for Barry's legal fund

– and the attention of John Nolte of Breitbart News Network – that Random House responded.

> False rape accusations are a serious matter. Lena Dunham and Random House allowed an innocent man to remain under a suspicion of rape when they knew the truth. This is a wrong that deserves correction. We have yet to hear from Ms. Dunham, who is the only person with first-hand knowledge who can truly exonerate 'Barry One's' reputation. It is unfathomable to us that she remains silent.

Then again, maybe he shouldn't have singled her out for criticism. After all, every other feminist remained silent on the matter, too.

IGGY AZALEA

Some celebrity feminists seem to have no idea what gender parity means.

So, when Iggy Azalea threatened to dismember her fiancé Nick Young over allegations of infidelity, she was – by the laws of equality – also saying it's fine for men to enact the equivalent revenge on their cheating girlfriends.

'You'll have half a penis,' she proudly warned her husband-to-be via a US radio interview. 'I already said, just one more thing and you will lose a quarter of your meat.'

Which, aside from being a vile threat of violence, is also a bit rich considering she'd previously chided Eminem for 'threatening young women as entertainment trend' (*sic*) and being a bad influence on his younger fans.

Pot, kettle, black – Iggy?

CATE BLANCHETT

As a grown woman in a free, civilised society, Cate Blanchett has every available opportunity to 'do a Diane Keaton' and attend red carpet premieres in a non-descript, androgynous trouser suit.

But, of course, she doesn't – because she clearly enjoys the glamour, beauty and sex appeal that come with the job. Not to mention the fact no actress has been denied a role because she scrubs up nicely.

So she's got something of a brass neck to scold show-biz journalists who acknowledge and respond to HER DECISION to wear an attention-seeking dress.

No doubt struggling to be heard over the swell of sympathy violins playing in the background, Cate originally voiced her first-world concerns as part of Amy Poehler's Ask Her More 'campaign', which lectured reporters by demanding they ask women the exact same questions as their male counterparts.

Er, except there's one crucial difference between the two men: on red carpets do not trade on their bodies in the same way women do. Therefore, Cate and her afflicted pals might want to control the outcome of their own experiences by making different fashion choices.

Thankfully, not every actress is so precious. Just look at the likes of Sarah Jessica Parker and Meryl Streep, who identify as all-encompassing 'humanists', rather than feminists.

When I met Damian Lewis's wife, Helen McCrory, at the launch of Alan Rickman's film *A Little Chaos*, she was equally clued-up on 'dressgate' when she said:

> If you don't mention what I'm wearing on a red carpet then I take a slight affront.
>
> I mean, I don't look like I'm going to the pub and it would be a bit embarrassing if everybody didn't look down and just said, 'So, how are you? We're just going to ignore the dress.'
>
> Part of the fun of it is dressing up and choosing something that people will say, 'What a beautiful dress.' I enjoy wearing it. Nobody's interested in what I wear off the red carpet because I'm not interested, so nobody else is either.

BAD EDUCATION

LONG BEFORE GREECE WAS THE financial dead-wood of Europe – destined, rather sadly, for life as a failed state – it was home to philosophy's founding father, Socrates.

A vanguard figure of education and critical analysis, his most notable students included Plato and Aristotle, who, between them, went on to establish the Academy in Athens (the Western world's first institution of higher learning) and teach Alexander the Great, no less.

Not bad, considering he started his working life as a stonemason.

However, this second-career success soon hit the skids when Greece's political climate changed and he found himself at the centre of a wacky legal wrangle. His crime? Questioning the status quo. Or, specifically, thinking outside the curriculum.

Tried and found guilty of impiety and corrupting the youth, he was sentenced to death by forced hemlock poisoning in 399 BC. Not exactly a high point of ancient history, I'm sure you'll agree.

But, rather than learn from this sorry state of affairs, we now seem doomed to repeat it as contemporary college campuses continue their own steady decline into batshit crazy.

Yep, rather than welcome intellectual diversity – which, BTW, is probably the single most important form of diversity, ever – many institutions now penalise independent thinkers for defying a new orthodoxy promulgated by the regressive left. Think I'm exaggerating? Think again (clue: that's the whole point of further education).

Spiked magazine recently conducted the second annual Free Speech Rankings, which highlight the scale of the intolerance problem. They found that 90 per cent of UK colleges stifle debate and alternative opinion if it doesn't reinforce the 'social justice warrior' narrative.

Unsurprisingly, this has ushered in a stalemate of 'safe spaces', restrictive language codes, trigger warnings, no platforms (whereby students disinvite guest speakers via protest) and frightful fancy dress bans. Even certain hairstyles are being outlawed (as I write this, YouTube footage of a young, white kid being harassed for his dreadlocks at San Francisco University is going viral).

And, apparently, it's getting worse, with the latest Spiked numbers showing a 10 per cent increase in campus illiberalism since their inaugural findings from 2015.

In particular, thirty institutions have blocked newspapers, whilst twenty-five expurgated songs, twenty banned clubs or societies and nineteen censored events. In addition, 42 per cent have censorious equality policies, 39 per cent have a no platform rule and a fifth have active safe spaces, some of which boast colouring books, bubbles and videos of frolicking puppies.

It's all very Orwellian.

The study's author, Tom Slater, was so perturbed by his findings that he went on to write a book called *Unsafe Space: The Crisis of Free Speech on Campus*, in which he says:

> The number one justification for this is that words hurt. This isn't just about snuffing out ideas they disagree with. They genuinely think that coarse, racist or simply un-PC speech poses a real and present threat. They equate

it with being punched in the face or being traumatised. That's a chilling shift. What's allowed this to breed is a lot of complacency from universities and liberals. The NUS' no platform policy, which bans racists and fascists, has been in place for over 40 years. Many liberals and university heads didn't challenge that. If anything, they nodded along. Now, the logic of no platform has spread, from fascists to feminists, from Islamist extremists to anti-Islamist campaigners. But this was inevitable. If you let censorship go unchecked, it will spread. That's the lesson of history.

But, hang on, where precisely did all hysteria this come from?

'Safe spaces originated out of the gay and women's liberation groups of the '70s and '80s, but they always had their problems,' Slater adds.

Back then, at the very least, the idea was that you had a space where people could discuss the challenges they faced and then come up with a plan to change things. They were seen as a means to an end. A stopgap before genuine liberation. Now, they're seen as the end. Hemming yourself in is the ultimate goal. That's really depressing.

As for trigger warnings, they started on internet forums for survivors of sexual abuse. The idea being to warn people about content in a post that might trigger traumatic feelings. Even on those terms, trigger warnings are problematic. Many psychologists say they actually stop those suffering from PTSD from facing their problems. But the way in which they've been expanded to cover experiences of racism, sexism, homophobia, etc., shows what a low view these campus types have of individuals. They effectively want to treat everyone as de facto mentally ill. Particularly if you're gay, female or black. It's patronising nonsense.

Agreed. So wouldn't it be easier to just write these over-zealous students off as the product of a generational blip?
'That's a cop-out,' he says.

They were raised in a society that has completely undermined free speech and moral autonomy. They were brought up on multiculturalism – not, that is, the diverse, lived experience we all enjoy, but the idea that it's culturally insensitive to challenge certain views. They went through a school system obsessed with anti-bullying, which taught them that anything that chips their self-esteem should send them running to the teacher. And they've grown up in a country that has criminalised so-called hate speech for decades. You don't have to look far to work out where they're getting their ideas from.

Even the elite schools have these problems. From Yale to Oxford, a growing number of student bodies are implementing their own totalitarian regimes, which are steadily destroying education from the inside out. Spiked's official rankings identify the worst offenders as Aberystwyth, the London School of Economics, Leeds, Edinburgh and Swansea, plus Birmingham, Birkbeck, Sheffield, Newcastle, Manchester, Oxford, Hull and UCL.

And, whilst this is alarming for anyone with a functional brain, these paradigm shifts are particularly worrisome for young blokes. Especially if they happen to be white and heterosexual, because this, critics claim, is the 'privilege' formula. One that instantly paints a bullseye on their backs.

Hence this chapter acts as a primer – or is it a reconnaissance mission? – for those who are about to embark on their own college journey. Because, whilst it was once about living away from home, cheap beers and the occasional all-nighter, it's now a minefield of censorship, character assassination and kill-joy conformity.

'When I was doing my research, the biggest revelation was how much the students' unions are overstepping the mark,' Slater adds.

> They're not just trying to censor students, they're trying to regulate their sex lives. I wrote a chapter about the campus war on lad culture – it's quite startling.

Mandatory sexual consent classes for rugby teams. Policies that stipulate how you can and can't chat people up.
It's creepy. And it's driven by a grim outlook – that men
are abusers-in-waiting and women are fragile flowers.

One man who knows this all too well is George Lawlor. He caused a ruckus in 2015 when, aged nineteen, he
refused to attend consent classes at Warwick University.

Justifiably offended, he respectfully argued that most
people 'don't have to be taught to not be a rapist' – and,
moreover, that predators probably wouldn't attend such
seminars in the first place.

Unsurprisingly, the reaction went nuclear. His picture was
splashed all over the national papers and he was driven out
of lessons with heckles of 'rapist' and 'misogynist', whilst
simultaneously being bombarded with violent threats online.

It got so bad that he became something of a recluse –
both socially and academically.

'Eventually, all the hatred and bile took its toll,' he
tells me.

By the end, it was difficult to get up in the morning and
I'd spend days resigned to my room. I didn't realise, but
I would often forget to eat, too. I just had so much on
my mind that it wasn't really a priority for me.

Of course, this all meant that my academic work

suffered. I missed whole modules and it won't be until the summer that I find out how this has affected my grades.

I lost friends too, but I suppose anyone willing to ostracise me for something so petty isn't worth knowing in the first place. I say good riddance. But I'm still worried about how the whole episode has affected my employment prospects.

My name and face are forever linked with the phrase 'rape culture'. A potential employer will always be concerned with perception and, in today's world, being perceived as something is almost as bad as actually being it.

Fortunately, amid all the madness, Lawlor did receive a modicum of moral backing from a selection of professors – which, FYI, isn't necessarily the norm. 'One was very good and reached out before anyone else. She was very understanding and offered me support. I really appreciated that,' he adds.

But where the university was adequate and, at times, quite helpful, the students' union was lacking.

'They are a political institution,' he continues.

I'm a right-wing libertarian, whereas they're infested with lefties, so we don't get on. Outsiders compare this to East Germany and describe the NUS as a 'student Stasi', but I think it's more apt to compare them with

France's court of Versailles. Campuses are bubbles, completely disconnected from the real world. They're ruled by absurd, fashionable ideas and those who don't follow them are quickly treated with disdain – or worse.

These people are in for a surprise when they graduate into the real world and find there are no safe spaces, but it worries me that they will later be the architects of society. Eventually, they will be the people to occupy the highest echelons of our government and other institutions. Let's just hope they open their minds before then or I fear today's campuses are the prototypes for tomorrow's United Kingdom.

Scary stuff, right? And this isn't even a Stephen King novel.

Not that this incident was isolated, of course. Simultaneously, 150 miles north, the University of York was U-turning plans for a modest International Men's Day meeting following melodramatic 'outrage' from – surprise, surprise – feminists.

This was despite the fact that, twenty-four hours earlier, a fellow student had killed himself and his death was the event's catalyst. Still, rent-a-gob gender warriors decided that young men responsibly discussing their collective issues without supervision might spark a campus coup.

In an open letter signed by 200 people (many of whom were former students or, even worse, incumbent lecturers), they declared: 'A day that celebrates men's issues – especially those outlined in the university's statement – does not combat inequality, but merely amplifies existing, structurally imposed, inequalities. Men's issues cannot be approached in the same way as discrimination towards women, because women are structurally unequal to men.'

It banged on:

> We recognise that patriarchy is damaging to both men and women. We do not, however, believe that the university statement engages with these complex issues with sufficient nuance or understanding. The failure of the Equality and Diversity Committee to do so undermines their self-proclaimed commitment to gender equality, and leaves us deeply concerned that their supposed investment in women's rights is mere lip service.

Like I said, batshit crazy.

Sure, people will say, 'Ah, you shouldn't judge feminism by this – it isn't representative of the wider movement,' but my response would be: BOLLOCKS! This absolutely TYPIFIES how modern gender activists behave. And, moreover, they're not insignificant fringe operators either. They're frequently heads of department and course leaders with influence and power (just look at the debacle in which university professor Melissa Glick was caught on camera asking for 'muscle' to remove a lone, dissenting student from a protest), which is precisely why we shouldn't dismiss them as harmless.

Another example is Goldsmith's former Diversity Officer Bahar Mustafa, who infamously used the hashtag #killallwhitemen on Twitter before banning white men from a student meeting. Thankfully, she was later forced to resign after allegations of bullying surfaced, but don't be fooled by this happy ending – her absence doesn't make academia any better for us blokes. There are plenty more where she came from.

Which, when you think about it, is a bit strange considering it has never been a better time to be a Western woman – especially in the gilded cage of university, where they outnumber men in their thousands and effectively run the joint (whilst probably smoking a few, too).

So where the hell does all this seething anger come from? And why does it seem to surface in equal, steady waves each year?

Wanting to avoid any conclusion-jumping, I approach Janice Fiamengo – resident English professor and all-round good egg at the University of Ottawa.

The motor behind this production line of pissed-off pupils, she says, is women's studies, a 'discipline' which seems intent on socialist indoctrination, rather than objective, fact-led education.

'Gender studies courses are the academic arm of the radical women's movement,' she tells me from her office on campus, which I'm assuming is reinforced for personal safety.

> Their sole purpose is to train young people to become activists for the feminist cause, and to take that commitment into their jobs in government, social work, journalism, law, and academia.
>
> As a whole, these programs are not about the pursuit of truth; they are about theories of oppression to be accepted rather than examined. Very few are interested in facts and evidence. They're about presenting a worldview in which patriarchal evil must be fought and heroic female victimhood defended.
>
> Students are taught, for example, that gender is a social construct without being given any assessment of the scientific evidence disproving such a fantasy. The emphasis is unremittingly on female grievance and supposed male privilege, never the other way around. Thus, students are given an entirely distorted view of their society, one that is entirely lacking in historical or cultural perspective.

In other words, they're radicalised.

This may sound a little sharp, but it's the truth. If

you look back at their history, these classes began at San Diego State University in 1970 after radicals demanded a female perspective on, er, facts. Which, by their very nature, have objective reality.

Predictably, the concept soon snowballed into a lucrative idea that was rolled out globally, helping to preserve the feminist rhetoric whilst monetising the movement and providing an illusion of intellectual legitimacy.

Yet, despite all this, it still doesn't have any academic rigour – which surely means it has absolutely no place in a university. Like voodoo. Not convinced? Just ask rising Rebel Media journalist Lauren Southern, who surreptitiously signed up to her local course (for research purposes only) at British Columbia's University of the Fraser Valley.

'It was basically a bunch of theoretical nonsense taught as fact,' she confirms.

> I would be hard-pressed to describe it as academic. In fact, it was scary how easily girls in large groups were coaxed out of intelligent discussion and into some emotional circle-jerk, devoid of reality.
>
> These students were not allowed to question the assumption they were oppressed – even if they wanted to. The whole course was shocking to me. Especially as the teacher put a gag on us discussing the syllabus outside of class, which I found very suspicious.

> For the sake of women, I would nuke the entire pro-
> gram. Not least because it was hardly about gender at all.
> That label was just a facade for Marxist indoctrination.

Disconcertingly, this listen-and-repeat dynamic is now a two-way thing, with college kids enforcing their own political mantra upon lecturers.

One recently penned an anonymous article for Vox entitled 'I'm a liberal professor, and my liberal students terrify me'. In it, he detailed how every uttered word is fast becoming a cause for dismissal. He wrote: 'Hurting a student's feelings, even in the course of instruction that is absolutely appropriate and respectful, can now get a teacher into serious trouble. I have intentionally adjusted my teaching materials as the political winds have shifted.'

Northwestern University's Laura Kipniss had a hard time after she questioned the exaggerated claims of campus rape. Her punishment for daring to fact-check? Not quite a pint of hemlock, but not far off. Incredibly, she was investigated under Title IX, which is a federal law used to fight sexual discrimination in education. That's right, people: a lecturer grilled by authorities over a dissenting opinion.

Since then, the wider situation has worsened, with a whole host of guest speakers blocked from making scheduled appearances. These include Warren Farrell (go online to see footage of teenage protestors in Toronto calling his seminar attendees 'rape-apologist scum'), activist Peter Tatchell, historian David Starkey and human rights campaigner Maryam Namazie – who students feared might criticise Islam, thus be racist. Even though Islam isn't actually a race.

Hilariously, even Germaine Greer and Julie Bindel have been blackballed from lecture halls, which, quite frankly, beggars belief.

'The left would have you believe that they're the tolerant ones, whilst claiming it's the right who are totalitarians with no diversity of thought – but the truth is the exact opposite,' says Dave Rubin, a man who – as the gay, liberal host of *The Rubin Report* – identified with the left all his life until they spectacularly lost the plot.

'My moment of awakening was the aftermath of the *Charlie Hebdo* attacks in Paris,' he adds.

> I was surrounded by people who were showing more sympathy for those who committed the crimes, rather than those who'd been killed. No matter how many times I tried to explain that there can be no excuse for murdering people over a cartoon, they turned it into how the perpetrators were the victims because the magazine's editorial staff didn't respect their beliefs.
>
> Not only is this a twisted perversion of reality, but it's

an incredibly dangerous game to play. What else should we not draw? What else should we not write? What else should we not think? Should we grant this veto over our thoughts and actions to any other group?

People are now afraid to post their own thoughts on Facebook because they don't want to be called racist or homophobic or anti-Semitic. That, in turn, hands the entire conversation over to the other side, who sweep in with supposed easy answers. This is the real danger of what this regressive, not progressive, ideology has done. It has silenced a huge portion of people who want to have honest debate about incredibly important issues. And the more people remain silent, the more power we hand over to the real bad guys.

Cheery stuff, I know. But, trust me, this is the little-known reality of modern university – and it needs to be told so that, at the very least, people enter into it fully informed.

So what else can young men expect when they access the sunny uplands of academia?

They should be prepared for a frustrating and potentially demoralising experience in which they will be told that their sex is responsible for all violence and oppression, that their masculinity is a curse they need to unlearn, that they're a threat to young women, that

they are 'privileged', had it too good for too long –
all undeserved – and that it's time they gave up their
unearned advantages and allowed their far more deserving 'sisters' a chance.

This from Professor Fiamengo, who, BTW, was once the
sort of victim feminist she now opposes.

In their classes, young male students will find that men's
role in building civilisation will be consistently denigrated, minimised, or outright denied, while the male
responsibility for violence, colonialism, rape, slavery, and
systems of oppression will be a regular theme.

They will be lectured continually about their pro-
pensity to rape and will be warned that all manner of
natural behaviors – from admiring a beautiful girl and
complimenting her to expressing an unorthodox opinion – may constitute discrimination or harassment. Any
sexual involvement whatsoever, even the most seemingly consensual, may be defined after the fact as sexual
assault merely if the girl decides that she felt coerced or
uncomfortable. The young man's life and career can be
ruined by her word.

My advice to young men at university is: document
all involvement with women; keep all emails and texts;
and don't ever have sex with a girl who's been drinking.

Blimey, it certainly doesn't sound like university is the Woodstock of a guy's education any more. Which begs the question: is college still worth the hassle?

According to the Organisation for Economic Co-operation and Development, the average UK undergraduate paid £6,000 in tuition fees for 2013/14 thanks to the government's decision to triple maximum fees. That's more than US and Japanese students, who paid £5,300 and £3,300 respectively over the same period.

As if this wasn't bad enough, the Institute for Fiscal Studies recently found that a typical student will now leave university with an average debt of more than £44,000. A burden they'll be saddled with until their fifties.

But, whilst they've become increasingly expensive to get, the value of these degrees has actually declined. Mainly as a result of sheer volume, but also because some dickheads now graduate with diplomas in David Beckham Studies (thanks, Staffordshire University).

Looking back at my own experience, which – in addition to an English degree – also gave me a beer belly and an overdraft, both of which took years to shift, I now realise that I could've achieved the same qualification through a distance-learning course whilst making inroads at a career-related job and earning money, thus side-stepping student insolvency altogether.

What I've also learned is that employers couldn't care less where – or what – you studied. Their only concern is whether you'll work hard or be a liability. And they'll base this solely on your achievements gained on their watch.

Fortunately, for the majority of us, the university of life remains the original and best. It's frequently a more intellectually stimulating, challenging and inclusive place. Not to mention cost-free and with a greater degree of credibility.

But what can be done for those who must go to university because they want to be barristers or doctors (and I don't mean the sort who buy their qualifications online like 'Dr' Gillian McKeith)?

'Combating these issues is difficult,' says Jonathan Taylor, the director of intervention initiative Boys and Men in Education.

> It requires tenacity and a steadfast spirit that refuses to back down. Success will not be achieved by any single event; it will be part of a process that will take years.
>
> The first step is to encourage voices – students, teachers, administrators, concerned parents, and so forth – to unapologetically speak out on behalf of men on campus. These groups would ideally begin by addressing local issues, and network among each other to address broader or more challenging issues as a team. There are

many other challenges that will arise along the way, but this is the first and most critical step.

Spiked's Tom Slater echoes these sentiments:

> So much of campus life is regulated now. SUs don't just want to ban speech, they want to regulate your sex lives and tell you what fancy dress you can wear. It's insane, but buck up. Students need to stand up to this.
>
> The time for toeing the line is over. Don't let anyone tell you wearing a sombrero makes you racist. Don't let anyone tell you Robin Thicke is triggering. Challenge them, criticise them, ridicule them. They've gotten away with spouting this nonsense for far too long.

Of course, George Lawlor recognises the importance of this, too. Not least because, at the risk of making a tenuous link, it's the fight Socrates himself didn't get to finish.

> I made headlines when I refused to attend that consent workshop. I made headlines again when the press reported how vicious the backlash was. These are what I am known for now. Relatively few people know that despite everything, I survived.
>
> They're not aware of the fact that I'm undeterred and will continue to say exactly what I want to say exactly

when I want to say it. As far as they're concerned, I tried that and my life was ruined by it. I would want to tell anyone, regardless as to whether or not they're a fresher, regardless as to whether they're male or female, to say whatever they like. Screw everybody else. Have whatever opinions you want.

If people don't like them, they'll let you know, but don't let that put you off. You'll survive and you'll be a better person for it.

Besides, what's the alternative? To let the lunatics take over the asylum? No, thank you. But that's the very clear and present danger. See, without free speech and independent thought, our once-wonderful academic institutions simply become institutions.

And who wants to find themselves in one of them?

HOW TO BE A
SUFFRAGENT

PEOPLE LIKE BEAR GRYLLS TELL us how to survive
ten days in the jungle, which is great and everything,
but let's be honest: how often do we find ourselves in
the rainforest with a moral dilemma?

Instead, the real wilderness is here and now. The
towns, suburbs and cities we live in – everywhere from

the boardroom to the bedroom. It's here, among the soft furnishings, where the really hard stuff happens.

For it is these places where little things determine daily reality, which then go on to create big cultural norms that shape our worlds. It's the theory of the butterfly effect applied to modern male experience.

In recent years, our discouragement from this has left a slow-burning loss over gain: we don't flinch as health, economic and academic success casually slips away. Which is unlike us. Throughout history we have always been on our toes – keen to protect our welfare. Ready to fight for survival.

That is, and always has been, part of our legacy.

Yet something about this has changed. A key component in our brilliance has stopped working. Since feminism became mainstream, part of our man-motor has understandably shut down. We've become apolitical about the core of our identity, which naturally means part of *us* is missing. We aren't operating to quite the same success formula as before.

Clearly, judging by the previous eleven chapters, this new configuration isn't working. In fact, at no other point in history have we needed to roll our sleeves up and muck in with man politics more. The future for our sons is bleak, not bright, on most fronts.

However, conscious masculinity is more than just

recognising these flashpoints as they hurtle towards you – possibly wearing earrings. It's also about responding fraternally. As a brotherhood.

This doesn't mean blind loyalty to all men at all times, not at all. Rather, it's about doing your bit for women, whilst ensuring they too fulfil their responsibility to good gender relations. You know, allowing fathers to see their children or not rinsing ex-husbands in a divorce.

Contrary to what people may say, this doesn't take anything away from women. It doesn't equate to fear or retro ethics. It isn't ungallant or mourning a patriarchal empire. Nor is it Twitter trolling, crying into your beer or being unsympathetic to the hurdles faced by wives or girlfriends in, say, the developing world. Oh – and it certainly isn't about the pendulum swinging too far the other way. If anything, it's about stopping it moving at all.

In a nutshell, this is what constitutes a Suffragent: someone who's part-gentleman, part-agitator in creating genuine, mutual balance whilst expecting respect for his own unique, valuable contribution as a bloke and, where necessary, laughing in the face of any bullshit which undermines it. Including Janet Street-Porter.

This, gentlemen, is the way forward. It's our best ever bet at finally finding workable solutions to the usual roll call of men's issues.

Naturally, it's all good stuff. It's adding to the merits

of every other trend that has helped upgrade the world into a more egalitarian and pleasant place. However, as with any change, it won't always be easy. Especially as it's rooted in power and politics: a deadly combination.

So, to help, here are the Ten Commandments – herein referred to as the Men Commandments – on how to be a stealth, and successful, Suffragent.

1) ACCEPT THAT IT'S ABSOLUTELY OK TO GET POLITICAL ABOUT BEING A MAN. THEN, YOU KNOW, ACTUALLY DO IT.

Offended by yet another newspaper headline? Bilious from bloke-bashing on British talk shows? Sick of hearing we're just a bit shit? Well, rest assured, that nagging feeling in the pit of your stomach isn't nausea from last night's curry, it's your brain saying: 'I AM POLITICAL STIMULI. RESPOND TO ME!'

Don't fear this. Politics is part of everyday life. Christ, even the Eurovision Song Contest is political, so, technically, we've got some catching up to do. Fortunately, the last person to win Eurovision was a man in a dress with a beard, so we're good at stepping outside conventional masculinity guidelines to make a point – and win. To push it forward, we simply need to apply this more strategically into the places where it's needed most: schools, homes, family courts, hospitals, charities and universities. You know, wherever we happen to be at the time.

Trouble is, because we're programmed to actively mistrust these instincts – men are protectors! women are the protected! – Suffragent causes can be hard to identify, so allow me to assist. Typically, for future reference, these are pretty much anything you instinctively know is a low blow: one that would erupt if the genders were reversed. If unsure, stop and ask yourself: Is this happening to women? Are they dealing with the same problem? Are they expected to take the same raw deal on the chin without good reason? If not, you're onto something.

Doing this is all about recognition. It's self-assurance that your perceptions are real, that the bullshit inequity exists and your hurt is justified. Feeling offended isn't a sign of weakness, it's a sign of self-respect, which is a strength.

Amazingly, joining the dots between other peoples' bloke-bashing and your misplaced man-shame is the first step in shape-shifting into a better version of yourself: it's like taking the red pill in *The Matrix*. Instantly, you realise the problem isn't you for just *being* a man. Instead, it's how the world makes you *feel* for being a man.

By getting political about this stuff, even just inside

your head, you're ring-fencing masculine identity and making it bulletproof. This is our protective instinct, turned inwards to help ourselves. Self-preservation meets stealth preservation.

In a dog-eat-dog world, this is crucial. It's also being socially erect, as opposed to flaccid, which makes you engaged with reality, not blindfolded from it. The consequence of this is that you maximise the odds of a good life on your terms.

If in doubt about embracing Suffragent status, consider this: Do you have a penis? Do you want to decide the fate of your foreskin? Would you like to determine when you become a father – if at all? Should your son survive school and have the chance of going to university? More importantly, do you want him to be proud of eventually becoming a man? And, likewise, do you want your daughter to instil the same values in her son?

Haha, of course you do. So congratulations: you're politically awake – and that's absolutely a good thing.

2) LEARN TO BE GOOD WITH YOUR TONGUE.

All modern men should be good with their tongues – and, no, I don't mean like that.

After years of ignoring our Suffragent cues, we can find ourselves with an under-developed voice on the big issues. So, it's crucial that we tone our mouths as well as our muscles.

A great, realistic place to develop this is the comments section of any online newspaper, which allows you to find your feet on topical issues privately, but publicly. Don't scoff; these forums can have genuine influence.

For a start it isn't emotionally throwing up in some Reddit thread or entering the black hole of a Twitter fight, which – as Ricky Gervais once said – is basically people shouting in a bin. Oh no, comment sections are different. They are postcards to the editor via the readers, which is exactly why every journalist obsesses over them. They are the ugly truth of public opinion and allow people to be heard.

They're also read by politicians, celebrities, authors and, more importantly, people who need reaching – men who feel disenfranchised or worn down. Perhaps even people who misunderstand us. Don't forget: people can't hear what we don't say. Disseminating a bit of rational, polite clout in these places has the possibility of mileage and influence.

For decades, male opinion (especially dissident male opinion) was nudged out of the media narrative to isolate it. The ability to reverse this, complete with an audience of millions, is reclaiming the right to being heard.

That aside, it's also a nice way to simply get something off your chest – a release valve that makes the media machine slightly more two-way, which is key considering how much it shapes our sense of self.

I once met a veteran female journalist who I can't name here because she'd sue me (and she can afford better legal representation than I can). When we met in Annabel's nightclub I told her that, having bought and read two of her books, I was disappointed that they often contained some pretty vile, undeserving stuff about men which made me feel shit – to the point where I binned the books in protest. Worse of all, it wasn't even *funny* stuff. I'd wasted hours of my life on something that didn't make me a) laugh or b) erect. What was the point?

At the time she said, 'I can't be held responsible for something I wrote five years ago. Besides, I've changed since then.' But, months later, after I began doing shifts on the newspaper she worked for, she penned another hateful piece claiming all men are sexist, sex-mad pigs. Naturally, I emailed her on the internal system and pointed out, with all due reverence, that she should try adopting a bit more empathy towards the opposite sex. Especially as we're all in this together, cheek to jowl.

Her response? She went straight to the managing editor and complained, ego in hand – how dare I, a man, especially a younger man – question her. I then got dragged into his office and had to explain myself – which worked in my favour when he revealed that, actually, I'd voiced the consensus of countless others in the building.

The one piece of advice he did give me, however, was also his wisest: that if I'm going to make a point, I should make it publicly – for others to see. This led me to my first men's issues column for MailOnline, which eventually formed the basis of this book.

Naturally, the said journalist's complimentary copy is in the post.

3) BURN YOUR BRIEFS.

Not literally, of course.

Instead, I'm suggesting you be a bit more like Chris Whitehead – the Suffragent equivalent of Billy Elliot. This young lad was just twelve years old when he wore a knee-length skirt to Impington Village College in Cambridge to protest his school's lopsided uniform policy, which randomly banned boys from wearing shorts during the summer.

This miserable bit of misandry may have been small-fry, but it meant lads had to swelter in classes for no reason, whilst girls were allowed weather-appropriate dresses – which, subsequently, affected concentration levels and a boy's ability to learn (office men subjected to suits in July, take note!).

Quite frankly, this was not cool, so he did something about it. Recognising everyday bullshit and vowing to change it, he addressed 1,368 pupils in assembly – rocking the skirt, I might add – and proved he had cognitive brawn as well as balls. The campaign was so successful it garnered support from Adrian Chiles, who wore a skirt on ITV's *Daybreak* in solidarity, and bagged a Liberty's Human Rights Award.

Four years on and this *still* makes me chest-swellingly proud. Not just because what he did was fuelled by fairness, but because he wasn't afraid to disobey old-fashioned rules about what men can do socially. This micro-rebellion is a crucial point because it rejects other peoples' stifling codes of behaviour, which often hold us back from addressing inequity.

Soon after his success, much like the closing scene in *Spartacus*, boys at other schools followed suit with copycat campaigns. Last year, seventeen lads at Whitchurch High School in Cardiff protested the same problem in skirts, forcing simple, common-sense change with a bit of intelligence and *humour*, which is also where it's at.

After all, there's no hard-and-fast rule saying these

things must be dry and dull. Us men are often brilliant at comedy, so let's use it for the last laugh.

4) GO YOUR OWN WAY.

Men are at the height of their personal power and bargaining position when they're single.

It's only when they give this away to girlfriends, wives and children (read: women they have children with) that they become compromised, so be aware of this before you sign it away.

Thus, when champion golfer Rory McIlroy called off his engagement to professional tennis player Caroline Wozniacki, it was a sign of real optimism for the male of the species.

In fact, if we ever needed to update the evolution of man diagram, from ape to human, the next incarnation might be his curly-haired silhouette with a ring-free finger, because – finally – a rich man realised that, sadly, marriage is often an expensive divorce-in-waiting. *Learn from this.*

Part of McIlroy's bitter pill was swallowing the reality that perhaps she didn't respect him quite as much he deserved. Just a few months before it ended, she posted an unkind picture of him sleeping – mouth open, dribbling slightly – online, knowing it would be picked up and published by every news agency in the world. OK, it was only a playful betrayal, but some would argue it was the distant relative of a kiss-and-tell or disclosing intimate sex details with friends over a bottle of wine.

Brilliantly, armed with the makings of a Suffragent brain, he clearly couldn't resolve this against his self-respect. So, rather than make an honest woman of her – which society says he must – he made an honest man of himself. Instead of shrugging it off and biting the bullet, taking it on the chin etc., he took the braver, more rewarding route.

Weeks later, it paid off: having won the British Open, he admitted the decision to stay unmarried made him a better, more focused golfer. He became his own best man without needing a best man, whilst she took to the press and, tellingly, said: 'At least I can date taller men now.'

Keep all this in mind if wedding magazines suddenly find their way into your home.

Men no longer get all the emotional validation they need from one woman, so they are more psychologically self-sufficient. As a result, men feel more deserving, less desperate to settle because that's exactly what they are.

The website dedicated to this 'go-your-own-way' phenomena defines such brilliant bachelor action as:

The manifestation of one word: 'No'. Rejecting silly pre-conceptions and cultural definitions of what a 'man' is. Looking to no one else for social cues. Refusing to kneel for the opportunity to be treated like a disposable util-ity. And, living according to his own best interests in a world which would rather he didn't.

In other words, it's saying I don't, rather than I do – which, funnily enough, has a very nice ring to it.

5) BECOME A FATHER, NEVER SOMEBODY'S BABY DADDY.

Traditionally, the natural progression, or common bedfel-low, of choosing whether to marry is whether to become a father. If the thirty-four years of putting my dad through his paces have taught me anything, it's that fatherhood is never, ever easy.

In fact, it's at least eighteen years of hard labour with a job description that combines teacher, doctor, social worker, entertainer, banker, removal man, therapist, driver and mediator, forever, without pay, whilst work-ing full-time and being told to 'do more round the home' by journalists with nannies. So it goes without saying that becoming a father should not be left to chance.

The rules are simple: do not become a parent unless it's something you absolutely, utterly want and plan. This isn't just a single, solitary decision you'll make once and never again – it'll need to be a religion you practise every time you have sex.

This sounds obvious, but I'm amazed at how many men sleep around without a condom, assuming their partners possess the same attitude to child-free life as they do – and always will. Perhaps these guys think it's rude to micro-manage their sperm during the heat of the moment, but this is mad considering nothing kills sex lives more than a screaming baby.

Don't be this guy. Even if it means you sometimes go home alone, WHICH IS ALSO OK. You do not need to sleep with every woman who offers you sex. In fact, the power in this is huge. Try it and watch your own stock rise.

Understandably, this can be tricky in the confines of a relationship – generally, you'll need and want to sleep with your partner on occasion (well, at least in the first few years) – but remember: when it comes to compromise, sperm is not something to be generous with. Women will not die without it. (OK, actually, we would *all* die without it – but not for a few million years, so relax. You are not personally obliged to top up the population, especially as it's already at breaking point).

If the decision to have a child with your other half ever reaches a stand-off, be alert to the value others place on those cheeky swimmers. I don't want to be as blunt as to say: 'Men, don't leave your sperm lying around', but men, please don't leave your sperm lying around, especially in condoms where it's preserved in handy packaging for people to use as impromptu self-insemination devices, because once your semen is off fertilising, your choices are fried.

Whilst you're at it, stop concerning yourself with ejaculation being premature and, instead, make it *mature*. Do this by embracing our oldest, most reliable survival technique: fear. This emotion normally means you're doing something potentially fate-changing. Of which sex is. Thus, treat sperm accordingly – with a healthy, respectful, life-affirming fear.

6) CONSUME THE MEDIA ACTIVELY, NOT PASSIVELY.

The media lies, constantly. The entire Leveson Inquiry was built on this fact, so mistrust everything that disses masculinity.

See, the media not only deceives, it also has an agenda and, currently, that agenda is to flatter women by making men look like perennial idiots.

This might seem good humour, but the constant drip, drip, drip can nag our brains into a sad, subconscious submission that works against us.

Looking back on my own experiences of media malaise, there was certainly a time when I *almost* believed I was worth less in society's eyes because I'm a man. I accepted women as better, more complex creatures because that message was so frequently asserted. Rather ironic considering how women used to be portrayed.

It was only when I allowed myself to see faults in all this and – in turn – question the messages underpinning musicals, computer games, talk shows, cartoons, novels and magazines – that I was eventually free of it. Try it yourself.

One of the best tips for instant relief is to avoid soap operas. Every single one of them portray men as weak and dishonest, whilst the women are all strong, stoic matriarchs. Sod that.

'Bad dads' in TV adverts is another one to avoid, but don't get angry, get analytical.

'Crap fathers are simply seen as an easy target, with broad enough shoulders to take blatant sexism in good humour,' says Jon Sutton, a chartered psychologist who blogs on parenthood.

But, when I look around, I actually see loads of dads doing a decent job. Sadly, I don't see this reflected in the press. I see them putting themselves down – with mums and the media doing the same. We internalise this and, as a result, the expectations of ourselves are lowered. It becomes a self-fulfilling prophecy.

Personally, I'm a big fan of the Bechdel Test applied to movies: Are there at least two women in the film? Do they talk to each other? Do they talk about something other than a man? It's amazing how few films pass this test, but I use a dad equivalent applied to supermarket ads. Is there a man in it? Is he a dad? Is he being anything other than a dick?

Find your own version of this and wear it like a visor.

7) BE YOUR OWN MINISTER FOR MEN'S HEALTH.

If there's one thing we truly need in order to succeed as a Suffragent, it's the minor matter of life itself.

Granted, this might sound a tad obvious, but considering we're forced to work harder at survival than everyone else, it's worth reiterating here.

Only recently a life-extending prostate cancer drug called Abiraterone was denied by the National Institute for Health and Care Excellence because it was deemed 'too expensive' at £100 per person – even though it potentially offers terminal patients an extra five years of life. Yep, that's how much you're *not* worth!

This isn't a cherry-picked case, it's proof of a culture where men die sooner so women live longer.

So, instead of holding your breath in anticipation of it improving – despite the fact nobody's actually paid to make it happen, such as a Health Minister for Men – commit to managing it yourself. Close your own life expectancy gap and those of the men you love. Be your own one-man army. Go to the gym (but to shift fat from around your middle, not to bulk up), keep tabs on the fags and the booze, live by the 5:2, don't go to work sick – stay home and rest – play Sunday-league football, vow to burn 1,000 calories each week, and chomp statins – or at least a daily aspirin, which thins the blood for better circulation.

Make your own bespoke health plan, too. Learn what issues affect the men in your family and identify ways to offset them. Take advantage of office gyms or workplace health policies. Try alternative therapies and combination supplements.

Then, take time to review yourself mentally. Regard it as a diagnostics check. Are you happy in life? Feeling OK? Depressed? Stressed? Once this is all clear, or cleared up, check others are also OK. Instil this kind of dual thinking in friends and family. From here, take it outwards. Suggest men-specific initiatives in your local health centre or school. Ask your GP surgery to open late for guys who spend all day in the office and can't make 9–5 appointments.

Then, take time to pressure your local care providers for details of what they spend across the gender lines. Get item-ised bills via Freedom of Information requests and share them on social networking sites. Give them to newspaper journalists and use humour to highlight the bias. This will further engage people.

But, ultimately, use healthcare sexism as your own per-sonal trainer. Imagine Mr Motivator meets Jeremy Hunt.

Then, ask the likes of Nicky Morgan, Minister for Equal-ities, exactly what she's doing about it all. She works for you, so ensure she justifies her salary.

Sometimes, understanding how little people care can be a life-saving catalyst in itself. This gives a whole new mean-ing to the term fighting fit. And, if you're going to fight, fight hard. Then win.

8) BE DISCERNING ABOUT FEMINISM.

Read that subtitle again, carefully. And once more, please. Clarity is essential here because what I'm asking you to do is be discerning about feminism, *not* equality. The two aren't necessarily synonymous and this isn't *Mein Kampf*.

Instead, at the risk of having faecal matter posted through my letterbox, I'm suggesting we apply some quality-control to a political movement which – for all its achievements and success stories – is still an ideology like socialism or Marxism and, like them, has followers on a spectrum of moderate to extreme.

Germaine Greer once said that women have no idea how much men hate them. Fortunately, we have countless examples of how much the sisterhood can despise us. Sadly, just as there are men's rights campaigners who are misogynists in moral drag, there are plenty of women who hate blokes with an irrational, catch-all passion – yet dress everything up as women's liberation, which is both classic denial and really bad PR for people who just want a level playing field.

After all, when a group of Muslims break off and become fanatical, the sane ones stand up and distance themselves. They preserve the credibility of their faith by discrediting radicalisation, which – let's face it – is never a good look, whatever the cause. Yet this never really happens with feminism. 'Killallmen' hashtags can trend on Twitter and nobody says anything. Jessica Valenti can wear 'I Bathe in Male Tears' T-shirts whilst ISIS slaughters men, but there's no outcry.

This is nothing new. Previously, feminism allowed the likes of Sally Miller Gearhart to suggest that 'the proportion of men must be reduced to and maintained at approximately 10 per cent of the human race', whilst even Jilly Cooper, queen of the bonkbuster, once said, 'The male is a domestic animal which, if treated with fairness, can be trained to do most things.'

Therefore, men who *aren't* discerning about feminism are turkeys voting for Christmas. Not because they're sexist, but because *people who call themselves feminists can be sexist*.

So, separate the good from the bad and be selective about what the movement offers. This way, when somebody such as actress Emma Watson gets up on a UN platform and declares feminism has been misunderstood by men, you'll know better.

Actually, we haven't misinterpreted it at all. We simply haven't forgotten the cruel bits.

Asking men to rewrite history here is absurd. Men shouldn't sign up for a movement whilst it tolerates people who despise them. OK, this might be a minority few – nobody knows for sure – but it's still real. So, if celebrities like Watson are going to patronise us with a random declaration that feminism is suddenly benevolent, she'll need to show key movement leaders disowning all the bile and pressing the re-set button.

This, gentlemen, is a deal-breaker.

As journalist Cathy Young wrote in *Time* magazine:

> Men must indeed 'feel welcome to participate in the conversation' about gender issues [as Watson said], but very few will do so if that 'conversation' amounts to being told to 'shut up and listen' whilst women talk about the horrible things men do to women, and being labelled a misogynist for daring to point out that bad things happen to men too – and that women are not always innocent victims in gender conflicts.
>
> A real conversation must let men talk not only about feminist-approved topics such as gender stereotypes that keep them from expressing their feelings, but about more controversial concerns: wrongful accusations of rape; sexual harassment policies that selectively penalise men for innocuous banter whilst ignoring women who do the same; lack of options to avoid unwanted parenthood once conception has occurred. Such a conversation would also acknowledge that pressures on men to be successful come not only from 'the patriarchy' but, often, from women as well. And it would include an honest discussion of parenthood, including many women's reluctance to give up or share the primary caregiver role.

Amen to that.

Even bestselling novelist Doris Lessing – one of the most celebrated fiction writers of the twentieth century, who became a feminist icon with hit book *The Golden Notebook* – said a 'lazy and insidious' culture had taken hold in feminism which revelled in flailing men.

'I find myself increasingly shocked at the unthinking and automatic rubbishing of men which is now so part of our culture that it is hardly even noticed,' she said at the Edinburgh Book Festival in 2001.

> Great things have been achieved through feminism. We have many wonderful, clever, powerful women everywhere, but what is happening to men? Why did this have to be at the cost of men? I was in a class of nine- and ten-year-olds, girls and boys, and this young woman was telling these kids that the reason for wars was the innately violent nature of men. You could see the little girls, fat with complacency and conceit whilst the little boys sat there crumpled, apologising for their existence, thinking this was going to be the pattern of their lives. The teacher tried to catch my eye, thinking I would approve of this rubbish.
>
> This kind of thing is happening in schools all over the place and no one says a thing. It has become a kind of religion that you can't criticise because then you become a traitor to the great cause, which I am not. It is time

> we began to ask who are these women who continually
> rubbish men. The most stupid, ill-educated and nasty
> woman can rubbish the nicest, kindest and most intel-
> ligent man and no one protests. Men seem to be so
> cowed that they can't fight back, and it is time they did.

Thus, take her up on the offer. Check facts, rather than privilege, and be logical: when you read news stories about the gender pay gap or domestic violence spikes during the World Cup, which – BTW – aren't true, question where this information comes from.

Then, prioritise making yourself well read, rather than well hung. Trust me when I say this will serve you much better in the long run.

Christina Hoff Sommers wrote two excellent books that remain culturally robust: *The War Against Boys* explains why the school system is allowing young men to fail, whilst her other offering, *Who Stole Feminism?*, looks at fact rather than distorted feminist folklore.

Esther Vilar's *The Manipulated Man* deftly explains the phenomena of being Under the Thumb – which no man should be, ever – whilst Dr Roy Baumeister's *Is There Anything Good About Men?* helps explain some brilliant forbidden truths: specifically, that men are fucking awesome. Other titles worth reading are Dr Helen Smith's *Men on Strike*, Warren Farrell's *Why Men Earn More* – plus his other title, *The Myth of Male Power*. Buy all of these and consume them because knowledge is power.

That said, having a healthy relationship with feminism (don't confuse total surrender and compliance with complete support) doesn't mean being suspicious of women. Most of the experts in this book are female and they are among our best advocates.

Feminism has certainly improved aspects of the world we live in for many women, but it is not perfect. It's also not the movement to address men's issues. The clue is in the name.

9) BUOY BOYS.

When author Hanna Rosin wrote *The End of Men*, even her young son got the hump – which says it all. The American journalist claimed men were on a one-way journey to the scrapheap, with women rising up the ranks to replace us in a new, utopian, female future. Yep, apparently we'd been blagging capability for centuries and those nifty technological/medical/industrial advances were just flukes.

Needless to say, it wasn't the happiest of reads. For those blissfully unaware, the polemic mainly involves

Rosin talking with other women – and a few nodding men – about the prospect of a bloke apocalypse, which surely can't be good for anyone, not least the women left behind to pick up the slack.

Thankfully, there was a happy ending, although not in the closing pages. Instead, it happened when her nine-year-old son saw the finished product and, justifiably offended, sent her a note saying: 'Only bullies write books called *The End of Men*.' Good lad!

To be fair, he had a point. Something attitudinal has certainly shifted with the perception of boys in recent decades – and it isn't good. Thirty years ago we were made of slugs, snails and puppy dogs' tails. Now, we're medicated for ADHD at twice the rate of girls.

In Nigeria, Boko Haram can set fire to a school dormitory killing fifty-nine sleeping boys – the third tragedy of its kind in just eight months – but we don't hear a peep from anybody important, including Michelle Obama, who's usually on red-alert with a marker pen, an A4 jotter and the White House Twitter account. Instead, we get radio silence and crickets. Yet, two months later when the same terrorist organisation kidnaps a group of schoolgirls, the world shows impressive unity and compassion, mounting a viral campaign in minutes. What gives? Why is boys' life worth less – or worthless?

Even Z-list personalities are getting in on the act. Josie

Cunningham – who, like a cast member of *Shameless*, infamously had a £4,800 boob job on the NHS to launch a 'career' as a glamour model – hit the headlines when she offered to abort her baby for reality TV bosses because it was a boy. Now that's shameless.

Obviously, this isn't to say that she's sexist because she's from an under-privileged background – such 'boycotting' isn't just a lower-class thing. Let me clarify now or forever have Owen Jones throwing copies of the *Socialist Worker* at me in the street. Actually, it's evident across all castes.

Esther Walker, the middle-class wife of Giles Coren, celebrity food critic for *The Times*, once wrote in the *Mail*: 'I know very little about boys, but what I have seen I really haven't liked. Boys are gross; they turn into disgusting teenage boys and then boring, selfish men.' She added that she'd 'die' if her baby was born male and claimed she was 'deeply, deeply suspicious of little boys', before describing them as the 'dreaded gender'.

Even the royal family felt first-hand the micro-aggressions of fashionable boy apathy. When Kate Middleton delivered Prince George, there was an audible groan from the left who clearly wanted another female monarch because we haven't had one for ... oh, wait a minute, never mind. One critic even used the word 'unfortunate' to describe this poor rich kid's arrival.

Gentlemen! This is a new low and, as former boys, it's our duty to sort this out.

As it stands, these kids are drowning, not waving. They're also being circumcised, vilified and rendered semi-literate in a school system in which white, working-class lads are the worst-performing demographic in the country. In fact, studies have seen school teachers actively underestimate boys' capabilities before they even start, with psychologist Michael Thompson declaring that: 'Female behaviour is the gold standard in schools, with boys treated like defective girls.'

This, we are told, is progress. But, if current trends continue, the last male student will graduate university – a place where men are now a minority group – in 2068. That's just five decades away.

Given that this has been repeatedly flagged up but remains unchanged, a cynic might say it was designed this way. That, perhaps, the resentment traditionally reserved for men has slid down the life continuum scale to boys, who are the target in a long-sighted plan to smash the patriarchy from the inside out – slowly making men an unemployable, uneducated underclass to redress the balance.

An elaborate theory or the truth? Who knows. But boys need intervention, both socially and academically, now.

Ask yourself: how would the world react if Hanna

Rosin's book was called *The End of Jews*, or *The End of African Americans*, or *The End of White-Collar Workers*, or *The End of Immigrants*, or *The End of Gays*? The world would go berserk. And rightly so. But men are all of these things too.

They are also the sum total of their combined experiences of youth, which is precisely why boys need buoying, not bashing.

10) STAND BY YOUR MANHOOD.

Men are brilliant.

Being a man is brilliant. Seriously, it is. We invented football, secret intelligence, beer, the internet, philosophy, architecture, cars, trains, helicopters, submarines and the aeroplane. Not to mention email, the jet engine, Polaroids, IVF, parachutes, electricity, solar power and remote controls. We developed modern medicine with the birth of anaesthetic. We've led all the industrial revolutions and sent rockets into space. We've fought in bloody wars with tin hats and bayonets – and *still* won.

The world we live in would be nothing without Alan Turing, Alexander Graham Bell, Sigmund Freud, Horatio Nelson, Winston Churchill, Ernest Hemingway and

Albert Einstein. Oh, and Jesus was a man. Assuming he existed, it doesn't get much better than that.

Oh – and then there's *you*. The most advanced, finessed version of mankind to date. So don't let anyone else tell you otherwise.

Currently, deconstructing men is every fucker's business. It is the fashionable fascism of a million different women – and many, many men. But don't be fooled. This isn't something we should ever adopt or partake in, because it's borderline self-loathing.

The driving force behind it all – the disposability of men across the board as thinkers, fathers, soldiers and leaders – is at the core of our issues and, like a game of reverse-psychology, keeps us locked in a cycle. In one way we want to prove our worth by overstating our utility as cannon fodder or cash generators. Yet, we also secretly believe the suggestion of worthlessness, so don't bother to challenge it – or the countless other issues that affect us. We don't believe we deserve to.

To counteract this you will need a zero-tolerance to stiletto sexism.

Trash TV guru Dr Phil himself nailed it when he said:

> You either teach people to treat you with dignity and
> respect, or you don't. This means you are partly respon-
> sible for the mistreatment that you get at the hands of

someone else. You shape others' behaviour when you teach them what they can get away with and what they cannot.

If the people in your life treat you in an undesirable way, figure out what you are doing to reinforce, elicit or allow that treatment. Identify the payoffs you may be giving someone in response to any negative behaviour. For example, when people are aggressive, bossy or controlling – and then get their way – you have rewarded them for unacceptable behaviour.

Because you are accountable, you can declare the relationship 'reopened for negotiation' at any time you choose, and for as long as you choose. Even a pattern of relating that is thirty years old can be redefined. Before you reopen the negotiation, you must commit to do so from a position of strength and power, not fear and self-doubt. The resolve to be treated with dignity and respect must be uncompromising.

And that, in a roundabout way, is how to be a Suffra-gent. It is a blueprint for modern men at ease with the personal occasionally being political.

From here on in, the rest, as they say, is up to you.

For although these words mark the end of this book, they also represent a potential new chapter of masculinity because, according to industry opinion, they shouldn't exist. Literary agents across London told me a product like this could never happen. *Should* never happen. That men don't complain, don't feel pain, anger or frustration, and that, even if they did, they were too restricted to do anything about it.

I was also warned that it would be professional suicide. That men wouldn't buy it and a 'feminist mafia' would label me misogynistic, ensuring I never work again.

Still, I did it anyway.

See, at the end of the day, none of this subterfuge really matters. Even if I'm sofa-surfing for the rest of my life, unable to pay the rent, this book will still exist and you will still have read it. If this happens with enough people to create even minor critical mass, or the smallest communal response, that is change in the making.

This humble connection – caffeine-driven words on paper and some willing, open minds – is the grassroots beginning of a potential revolution. Perhaps even the ultimate game-changer.

What's genuinely exciting is that it *is* possible. There really can be a future where all the conundrums of contemporary masculinity are solved because the solution is already within us.

After all, we are brilliant. We always have been and we always will be. Then again, you already know this.

But this means absolutely nothing unless we stand – chest out, shoulders back – by our manhood.

ACKNOWLEDGEMENTS

FIRST AND FOREMOST, THANK YOU to Iain Dale for his vision, courage and belief. Oh – and for the advance.

Special gratitude to the entire Biteback Publishing team, especially James Stephens, Phillip Beresford, Suzanne Sangster, Sarah Thrift and my editor, Olivia Beattie. This book found the perfect home.

Heartfelt thanks go to my parents, Jean and Peter, who – along with my gorgeous/intelligent/inspiring sisters, Jane, Beth and Jenny – have always been brilliantly supportive,

STAND BY YOUR MANHOOD

even when I had bad hair and a brace. Apologies once again for that awkward adolescence. I love you all.

Ditto to the kids and in-laws – Evie, Natasha, Luke, James, Andrew, Jason and Andy – plus those I can no longer thank in person: Uncle Al, Uncle Jim, Jimmy Mac, Nancy, Peggy, Nog, Jean, Dinah and Anna.

Additional credit goes to each of the experts I interviewed along the way, plus the entire editorial team at the *Mail on Sunday* and MailOnline, including: Geordie Greig, Charlotte Griffiths, Barney Calman, Sarah Hartley, Andrew Pierce, Louise Saunders, Barbara Guiney, Anna 'Hurricane' Hodgekiss and, most notably, Deborah Arthurs, who first allowed me to have a voice.

I am also beholden to Brian Viner for *that* *Book of the Week* review, Kelly Ranson for her time-buying assistance and the glamorous *Daily Mail* books department for their kick-ass serialisation: Sandra Parsons, Susie Dowdall, Sally Morris and Julia Richardson.

I'd like to tip my hat in the direction of Gordon, Jane and all at Graham Maw Christie.

I'm also grateful to James Eppy, Lucy Pullin, Emma Dally, Richard Ehrlich, Tim Sigsworth, Hannah Hope, Sean Smith, Matt O'Connor, Erin Pizzey, Paul Elam and, of course, Luke, for the crucial introduction.

Last, but not least, a special thank you to my best friend, Bill.

I'd like to take this opportunity to formally honour the men in my family who died serving their country in the First World War:

Leading Seaman George Alfred Flood

Private Frederick Edward Cartwright Flood

Lance Corporal James Wood Hanson MM

Private Thomas Wood Sanders